Injustice
OF
Infertility

A TRUE STORY OF HEARTBREAK, DETERMINATION AND NEVER-ENDING HOPE

JENNIFER ROBERTSON

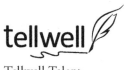

Tellwell Talent
www.tellwell.ca

ISBN
978-0-2288-3621-6 (Hardcover)
978-0-2288-3620-9 (Paperback)
978-0-2288-3622-3 (eBook)

DEDICATION

To the warriors who have been touched by infertility. This isn't a club we would ever choose to be part of. But together we can stand strong, and give infertility the bird.

TABLE OF CONTENTS

PREFACE

For the woman who is suffocating in her need for motherhood, yet cannot grasp it in her hands. Who feels a little piece of herself die each day and cannot recognise the person she has become. Where her first thought each morning is having a baby, and who cries into her pillow each night because it didn't happen today.

I am truly sorry that you have to go through this. You have done nothing to deserve this, and more importantly, this is not your fault. I wish I could take your pain away and turn back the hands of time before you realised that sometimes life doesn't go according to plan. Before your fairy-tale was destroyed and you were told that Santa Claus doesn't exist. But I can't do either of those things and nor can you.

Instead of looking backward, or sideways, I encourage you to keep your head held high and your eyes forward. Don't give up on life just yet. This may be a long and painful road, but I have learnt that we can endure more than we ever imagined possible. Your happily ever after will come. It just may not be according to your timeline or the picture you had in your head. The key to everything that happens on this journey from here on, is inside you. This is the fork in the road. You can give up on life, throw your hands up in the air and walk away. You can blame yourself and those around you, and get consumed in anger, jealousy and the injustice of it all.

Or you can put down that bag right now; you can take back the control that this disease has stripped from you, and you can keep putting one foot in front of the other. You can wake up each day, tell infertility to F-off, and not allow it to consume you.

This book is for me just as much as it is for you. So, strap yourself in – we're going to ride this fertility roller coaster together.

Chapter 1

WHERE IT ALL BEGAN

nfertility was not my first rodeo - but it was the first bull I ever rode that bucked me off and laid me on my ass. It broke me open and created scars that never really healed.

I hate admitting that because I've always prided myself on being such a strong person. I was the glue that kept people together. The sensible or sane one. Always practical and very pragmatic.

But over the next ten chapters, I'm going to be completely open and honest with you. Hell, for the first time, I'm going to be honest with myself. Because I have denied how much my fertility journey affected me for way too long. I was so focused on convincing everyone else around me that I was ok, that I, in turn, tricked myself into believing that I was too.

It became apparent, however, when I found myself sobbing uncontrollably while writing my story, that I had not grieved, dealt with or realised how much it had impacted me.

Before you join me on this journey however, you need to know about the woman I was before it began.

My strength and my need to be perceived as strong started when I was a little girl and escalated as the years went on. When I was five years old, my parents separated. To be honest with you, I don't remember a lot about it. I'm the youngest of three girls, so perhaps I was sheltered from it a little. Or maybe I blocked it out?

After they divorced, my mum and dad did their best to remain on speaking terms, so we weren't caught in the middle of the firing line. Above all, I always felt loved. Every Sunday night we would chat to our dad on the phone, and on school holidays he would hop on a plane to visit us. We were as close as you could be considering we lived 2,500 kilometres or 1,500 miles apart. He was quiet, had a wicked sense of humour and a short fuse. He had a heart of gold, was extremely loyal to his friends, dedicated to his family and loved us more than anything else in the world.

My mum was and still is a very strong-willed and determined woman. She was strict and had high expectations. At the time she was fiercely independent and set in her ways. She was completely driven and could do anything a man could do, but better. Paint a house, change a tyre and grow the lushest lawn on the street. I thought she was superwoman. She didn't need a man to survive. In fact, it became apparent over the years that she was better off without one.

I learnt about money pretty quickly when we were growing up. We would ride our bikes to school each day because we couldn't afford to fill the car up with petrol. There were no luxuries or treats, except on our birthdays. I was so conscious of the fact that we didn't have much money, that on the days we were allowed to buy our lunch at school, I always selected the chicken drummies over the meat pie. I really wanted that meat pie, but I didn't ask for it, because I knew it was more expensive and would stretch the budget too much.

My mum prided herself on the fact that she never put her hand out for child support payments from my dad. I think she was so determined to prove that she could do it all by herself, it would have killed her to take a hand-out.

The one extracurricular activity we were allowed to participate in outside of school was ballet. My dad paid for lessons for all three of us girls, and from then on, our entire childhood revolved around dancing. We spent every afternoon at the ballet studio. We performed in concerts and competed in dance competitions across the state for the next ten years. In the beginning, I loved it. I was good at it too. Medals and statues of ballerinas filled our trophy cabinet at home. My mum would spend hours sewing costumes, and when it was competition time, we'd park the cars on the street and practise our routines in the carport over and over again. On reflection, I hated the competitiveness and the pressure. In the lead up to competitions and exams, I'd have bad dreams and would feel sick from nerves. My need to be the best and the requirement to be perfect, from every pirouette to the way my body looked, started to overtake everything. I punished myself if it wasn't perfect. I wanted to please everyone around me from my teacher to my mum. I just wanted to make everyone proud of me. In the end, however, it became unenjoyable. The steps were harder, the stakes were higher, and I didn't like the fact that I wasn't the best anymore.

After I'd been dancing for around five years, I joined another dance troupe. We used to sing and dance and perform at shopping centres and community events. I loved it because there was less focus on perfection, I wasn't up there by myself, plus we were jumping around and dancing to pop music. For the better part of my puberty, I grew up performing. Being in the spotlight, there was always pressure to be perfect – the perfect body, the perfect make-up, the perfect hairstyle. But it wasn't as intense as ballet, and I loved the social life.

At school, I considered myself completely average. I was painfully shy and had a small group of friends. I tried to fit in and not stand out. I found out that you were criticised if you wore different shoes or weren't sporting the coolest backpack. Of course, my mum didn't care about the cool stuff, nor could we afford it. So, I spent most of my school years trying my best to blend in with the crowd, using the tools I had.

I wasn't naturally smart. You know those people who just understand concepts and pick things up easily? That wasn't me. I achieved good grades, but I worked my ass off to get them. When I was in year 10, my dream was to be a hairdresser. At the time, I was working as an intern at a hairdressing salon, and they had just offered me an apprenticeship. I was all set to quit school and start cutting hair. Except I hated the work. I was so shy and quiet and found it hard to talk to customers.

Around this time, we had a teacher in our dance troupe who was an accountant. Her name was Amanda, and she was beautiful, smart, poised and wore the best suits and shoes. I idolised her and wanted to be her. And when I found out how much a hairdresser earned compared to an accountant, I changed my mind. I never wanted to be poor or struggle with money. So that was that. A quick decision – I was no longer going to be a hairdresser; I was going to be an accountant, just like Amanda.

My two older sisters had a lot to do with my drive and determination. I looked up to them and idolised them. They seemed so much smarter than me and were always doing things that I wasn't allowed to do. If they shaved their legs, I wanted to shave mine. If they went to a teenage party, I begged my mum to let me go too. But my mum was very strict and had a whole lot of rules which seemed unfair at the time, but were completely reasonable (well, most of them). I wanted to grow up quickly so I could keep up with my sisters. They were moving out of home and getting jobs and travelling, and I wasn't moving anywhere. I felt like I was competing with them for my mum's praise. I didn't want to disappoint her, so I pushed harder.

At school, I studied hard and got into university. I hated university. I hated studying. I hated the pressure of an exam situation. It would make me feel sick with nerves. I used to put so much pressure on myself, and because I had to study my ass off to pass, I was always disappointed with my grades. I never failed any subject, but I didn't do as well as I wanted to. I was an average student. And I found out very quickly that I don't like being average. I am indeed a perfectionist by nature.

It was around this time that I fell in love. His name was Alan, and we met at a nightclub when I was sneaking into clubs at 17. He was good looking and a real charmer. At that stage, I was completely inexperienced in love and anything to do with the opposite sex. I felt awkward around boys. Hell, I felt uncomfortable around anyone. Sure, I'd had a couple of boyfriends before that, but nothing too serious. I was still a virgin at the age of 18, which was a foreign concept back then. I felt the pressure to lose it and keep up with my sisters and the rest of my friends, so with a little courage under the influence of alcohol, it happened. I hated it, as I'm sure most do on their first time. But I felt like a woman, and now I was hooked to this boy. He was very outgoing, so he was someone I could hide behind.

We dated for the next three years, and our lives became intertwined. His parents just so happened to own an accounting firm, the same accounting firm in fact that

Amanda had worked in four years earlier. I know, right?!! So, I got a job with them, and Alan and I moved in together.

And then my world fell apart. He broke up with me, and I had no idea why. He had become such a big part of my identity by then that it stripped me bare. I had no idea who I was without him. I was a complete mess. I look back at the person I was then, and I am deeply ashamed. I was lost, weak, needy and would have done anything to get him back. I lost a lot of weight and went out drinking with friends to drown my sorrows. I begged him to take me back. He treated me like a piece of shit, but I took it. In hindsight, he just wanted me to leave him alone, and I wouldn't. I would repeatedly text him (yes, drunk texting), and drive to his house to see if he was home. I guess you could call it stalking.

I wish I could go back to that young girl and shake her shoulders and tell her that she's better than that. It's like she is someone else – a young naïve little girl that I feel so sorry for. I'm embarrassed at how dependent I was on a man and hated how powerless it made me feel.

At the time, I was 21 and floating completely directionless, so when Alan's sister suggested we go on an overseas Contiki tour to Europe, I said yes. In the months leading up to our big trip, we booked tours and started getting excited. Despite my deep state of depression, it gave me something to look forward to. I don't know whether it was the fact that I was focused on other things, but just before we hopped on the plane, Alan had a change of heart.

He wanted me back. And I jumped at the chance to put myself back together.

I kissed him goodbye before I boarded our international flight, excited at what lay ahead. Not only Europe - but life in general. I'll be honest; I don't remember a lot of the trip – I drank my way through Paris, Switzerland and London. But I loved the sense of achievement and independence it gave me to travel to different countries and see the world. I felt a bit of strength come back and found a little piece of me again. And strangely enough, I didn't miss Alan at all.

When we arrived home, he was waiting to collect us from the airport. He proposed to me in the airport car park. I was shocked, and to be honest, I felt a little bit sick. I asked him if I could think about it. He said no. So, I said yes. In that split-second decision, my life took on a whole new direction.

Our lives intermingled once more, and I lost myself again. We moved into a house next door to his parents, and I received a promotion at work.

The only part of my life at the time that wasn't consumed by him, was cheerleading. Yep, in the short few months that Alan and I had broken up, I had caught up with an old friend from dancing who was cheerleading for the local basketball team. She invited me along, and that started new friendships and a whole new outlet for me. An outlet that would eventually become my safety net.

Two years later, Alan and I got married. I remember sitting in the hotel room with my girlfriend the night before my wedding, feeling complete dread. There was no laughter or excitement, just foreboding. I was still so insecure, and there were rumours that Alan was being unfaithful. Actually, there were rumblings the whole time we were together, but I pushed them away and turned a blind eye. My intuition told me it was true, but I had no idea how to create a new life for myself. I was so worried about what people would say about me if I didn't go through with it. So, I took the easy way out. The next day I walked down the aisle and married him. Despite my better judgement, despite knowing that he wasn't the one for me, despite knowing that I wasn't happy.

I hated being so weak. I hated being paranoid. I hated being jealous. I was also scared of history repeating itself, given the fact that my mum had been married and divorced previously. She was the strongest person I knew, but in relationships; well, she sucked. I didn't want that to happen to me. I was afraid of going down the same path, so I pushed on and kept up the facade.

We purchased a block of land and built a house together, because that's what you do. And then it happened. He started having an affair. I have no idea how long it went on for, but it was the ultimate betrayal. I was understandably devastated and angry, but the most surprising emotion I felt.......... was relief. I finally had a way out where people wouldn't judge me. I could walk away and not feel like a failure. I was able to push all of the fault and all of the guilt onto him. Because if there's one thing I hated most, it was failing. Failure was not an option.

We got divorced before our 2nd wedding anniversary. There was no negotiating or couples counselling. I had made up my mind and didn't need to hear his side of the story. I walked out of our house the night I found out about his affair, and I never went back. He called me cold and heartless. But I didn't care. I had made a mistake to take him back before, and I was never going to put myself in that position again.

So, this little caterpillar became a butterfly. I shed my cocoon and decided that I would never allow a man to take over my life again. My cheerleading girlfriends gave me the confidence, encouragement and support I needed to get back in the game. We partied, we danced, we cheered, and I made up for all the time I had lost. I went from someone who, at the age of 25, had only had sex with one man, to Samantha in Sex and the City. Ok, maybe not that wild. But I had been cheated on and felt utterly humiliated and betrayed. So, I set about proving that I was, in fact, desirable and men were disposable.

Not the healthiest way of dealing with things, but it was a lot of fun!

Shortly after, I quit my job at the family accounting firm and started a new role at a larger firm. After working there a while, a girlfriend was moving to the city and invited me to go with her. At the time, I was floating. I knew I wanted to focus on my career and get out of the small town I was living in. I had no desire to settle down and have a family just yet, and the options for promotion where I was working were limited. So, along with a few other girlfriends, we packed up and moved.

Going from a small town to a big(ish) city was a refreshing change. I got a job with a global accounting firm on the 25th floor of a high-rise building, right on the river. I loved the hustle and bustle of working directly in the city. Walking down the street in my high heels and power suit along with a million other workers, being anonymous was utterly empowering. I became Miranda from Sex and the City now. Yes, I was obsessed with this show!

I worked my ass off and partied just as hard. I was good at my job and pushed for promotion after promotion. After a few years, I bought an apartment and lived in a complex with some other girlfriends. I prided myself on achievement. I would look back on where I started – in a small town where I was weak. A place where the only thing to do was settle down and have kids, to being a manager at a corporate accounting firm and standing on my own two feet in a big city.

Around that time, my dad was diagnosed with cancer. He didn't tell us until after he'd had surgery to remove his kidney because he didn't want to worry us. So, it wasn't real until the cancer came back again. I had no idea how to process his illness, so I pretended that it wasn't happening. Until it became very real. He was undergoing chemo, so I jumped on a plane and flew to see him. He was the same old dad, with the same sense of humour, but there was a slowness, a foreboding that surrounded him. It was like he had given up the fight and was just waiting for the end to happen. We never spoke about his illness. It was like the elephant in the room. But I couldn't face the conversation or ask him whether he was scared. I was trying to be as strong as I could for both of us. I don't remember crying until I said goodbye and got on the plane to come back home. The tears slowly fell down my cheeks, and a heaviness settled on my chest.

When the plane landed at home, I was met with several text messages from my mother. My nanna, who lived 30 minutes away from me in the next suburb, had taken a turn and was in the hospital. There was talk of cancer and organ failure, and my mum was crying at the end of the phone, telling me that I needed to get to the hospital quickly. So, I caught a taxi home, dropped my bags in the front door and drove as fast as I could to the hospital. I sat with my nanna and held her hand for hours. She was fine when I had left to go and visit my dad, but now she was lying in a hospital bed, talking to me as if she was saying goodbye. I loved going over to her house and spending time with her. She would tell me stories and chat away without requiring a response. I found peace in our visits.

The nurse came in and told me that I could go home and get some rest. I must have looked like hell by then. I kissed my nana goodbye and told her I'd be back in the morning. At 8 am the next morning I received a phone call from my mum and through her sobs, I learned that my nanna had passed away.

This was my first real experience with grief. But I never got a chance to sit in it. Soon after, we got the news that the chemo wasn't working and my dad's cancer was terminal. By then, I was a complete mess and had huge regrets. I should have visited him more often. I should have called him more often. I was lucky enough to have a fantastic boss at the time who was able to organise a transfer with work to an office which was an hour away from where my dad lived. So, I packed my belongings in my car and moved to help care for him.

Watching someone you love slip away and being completely powerless to stop it is heart-breaking. It's soul-destroying. But I closed it all off. During the day I would go to work, and at night I cried in the safety of my makeshift room in the garage. Despite his diagnosis being quite clear, I still never asked him how he felt about it. Was he scared of dying? Did he have a good life? Had he done all the things on his bucket list? I never asked the questions, because I was so scared of the answers. I didn't want to take that lid off. I didn't want him to see me cry, and I didn't want to show that I was breaking apart. So, I pushed it down and kept pretending that I was strong.

Two months after my nanna passed away, we buried my dad. I saw him take his last breath. I held his hand as life slowly left his body. And I was the one who called my sisters and told them that he had passed away. I put on a brave face, and people commented on how strong I was. They admired my strength and bravery. So, I took on that role. I was the strong one who pushed through, no matter what.

In the lead up to and after dad's funeral, there was a constant stream of family and friends. As an introvert, that's hard enough; however, I was also trying extremely hard to keep a lid on my emotions and support everyone else. I craved warmth after waking up every morning with ice on the windshield of my car. At the time, I blamed it on the miserable weather, but I was freezing from the inside out, and my body was rigidly tense from holding in all the emotion.

I was exhausted from trying to outrun my grief and desperate to find a safe place to release my emotions without anyone seeing me break. So, I escaped to a tropical island, in the South Pacific Ocean, alone. I would wake up each morning and head down to the breakfast buffet; then I would move to lay by the pool, then go back to my bungalow for a nap, then come back down to the restaurant for dinner and read my book. I think the other guests and staff thought it was odd that I had come to one of the most romantic island resorts by myself. However, it created enough space for me to stop imploding and recharge just a little.

I thought that if I spent a week "grieving", I could leave it all behind on the island and come home without the baggage. The thought makes me smile now at my complete ignorance.

THAT is not how grief works. I know that now.

Have you ever noticed that no one ever congratulates you for crying and being vulnerable?

When I came back from my "grief holiday", people complimented me on my strength and courage.

And given the fact that I am an overachiever, I prided myself on the fact that I am strong, I am brave, and I can get through anything.

After I got divorced, I used to have nightmares that I would go back to being that weak, desperate little girl who got married out of fear. The one who allowed herself to be mistreated, humiliated and taken advantage of.

As a result, I created a new way of approaching life and a stronger version of myself. I was determined and was quick to make decisions. It was either black or white.

If you hadn't noticed yet, I am indeed your typical Type A personality. I am impatient, I search for efficiencies, I crave a sense of achievement, I despise laziness, I have an overactive mind, I'm ambitious and if I say I'm going to do something – I will. Some would call me stubborn or even pig-headed.

I learned from my upbringing and experience over time, that hard work equals results. The harder you work, the better the outcome. That's how my life had gone. I studied hard at school = I got good grades, I studied hard at university = I got a good job, I worked hard = I got a promotion. And to be honest, up until that point, this approach had worked just fine.

I ticked all the boxes and my process for getting through shit situations had worked. I faced things head-on – bring it on bitch!

Up until now, I had basically strong-willed my way through every situation that had come my way.

But infertility was bigger than anything I had faced before.

Infertility was a beast.

It started an unravelling of monumental proportions and turned everything that I had believed in up until that point on its ass.

Chapter 2

THE CREATION AND CRUMBLE OF OUR PICTURE-PERFECT PLAN

I've always had a clear picture in my head of how I wanted my life to turn out. I wanted the fairy-tale. You know, the one where the knight in shining armour on his white horse sweeps the princess off her feet? They fall madly in love, get married, have children and live happily ever after.

But here I was, 25 and divorced. The rug had been completely pulled out from underneath me, and the ground I was standing on was now completely unstable. I was lost, alone and floating directionless. Not only that, but the thought of trying to put the pieces of my life back together again and start my fairy-tale from scratch was daunting, and I was already so tired. Everyone around me was moving forward, and I was afraid of being left behind.

It felt like I was sitting at a crossroad, not sure what to do next. Zero plans. I no longer trusted myself to make the right decision given the mess I had created of my life so far. I needed clarity and an answer to the question that was keeping me awake at night. *Would I get my fairy-tale in the end?*

And this is how I ended up in the front room of my sister's house, sitting across from a psychic, hanging off her every word. I didn't care that she was a stranger. It didn't matter whether it was bullshit or not. I wanted her to tell me what was going to happen next. I needed her to reassure me that everything was going to be ok.

My first question? How many children would I have of course! Not whether I would, or how it would happen, but the quantity. When I ran that dream scenario in my mind, how many children should I be picturing frolicking in the back yard behind the white picket fence?

It didn't occur to me that it might not be a possibility. It didn't cross my mind that the question I should have asked was IF I would have children, or how long it would take, or how the journey would progress. I look back at that young, sweet 25-year-old with complete love and a little envy. So innocent and naïve, with no idea of the path that lay ahead of her.

The psychic told me I would have three children from two pregnancies. My mind went wild with possibilities.

Would I have twins? Would I marry a man who already had one child? I had a picture in my head of how things would turn out, and I completely indulged in the news. I trusted her implicitly because she told me exactly what I wanted to hear, and it gave me hope. I walked out of the session with a little more direction and purpose, knowing that life was going to be ok. Today that memory remains with me and makes me chuckle a little, knowing the way things turned out in the end.

I spent the next five years forming amazing friendships, travelling, partying and working my way up the corporate ladder. I excelled at single life. While my girlfriends were continually searching for love, I was doing everything I could to repel it. Every time it got close; I ran in the other direction. I loved having control over my life, and I was scared at the prospect of losing myself inside a relationship and getting hurt once again.

But after I turned 30, something switched for me. I was unfulfilled. The walls I had built up around myself for protection were closing in. I missed the companionship and someone to share myself and my life with. I was sick of being so strong and independent and wanted someone to take care of me for a change. I craved romance and true fairy-tale love. I realised that I was lonely.

That realisation started something else that I hadn't felt before. My biological clock started ticking. Looking back now, it seems absurd to be worrying about your childbearing years slipping away at such a young age. But, according to google, you're most fertile in your mid-20's with it declining in your early 30's, and declining even faster after you reach the age of 35. Ouch!! No wonder I was concerned.

But lucky for me, I finally met a guy.

Our eyes met across a crowded room, the background noise disappeared, the crowd blended into the distance, and it was love at first sight. Queue a cheesy Backstreet Boys soundtrack into the mix for full effect.

Just kidding!

The man of my dreams wasn't knocking down my front door, and being the impatient person I am, I knew if I wanted something to happen, I had to do it myself. So, I joined the online dating world. All my girlfriends were doing it, and from their stories, it sounded entertaining. I also needed to be in control of the situation because the thought of putting myself back out there again was terrifying. So, I did up my profile, posted it, and filtered the crap out of my applicants. Yep, I squeezed as much emotion out of it as possible. I approached the process of finding a man with all the romance of a job offer.

He was the first profile to make it through my filtering process. His name was Craig, he loved travelling, spending time with friends and family, his favourite film was Shawshank Redemption and he could construct a sentence. Tick, tick, tick. He was cute, entertaining, and most of all, he made me laugh. So, after our first date, we went on another one, and then another, and another. He had great friends and a beautiful family. I could see myself building a life with him and having a family together.

From the very beginning, we were upfront with each other in terms of our desire for children. We both came from families where children were a large part of the equation. I saw how he loved his nephews and how he played and interacted with my niece and nephew, and I knew he'd make a great dad. So, we didn't look back.

We spent the next two years travelling, dreaming and planning our life together. I still look back on those years fondly — such amazing times. There was no stress about IF we would have a family. We had our white picket fence life laid out neatly in front of us. We both wanted at least two children and were organising our life accordingly.

We spent six months searching for the perfect place to raise our family. At the time, we were living in a two-bedroom inner-city apartment. This didn't match up with the picture I had in my head of my children jumping on a trampoline in the backyard, while Craig and I looked on from the back deck with pride.

Eventually, we found and moved into our family home. It had a big yard, was close to the water, parks and some excellent schools. And it even had a white picket fence!

Craig and I would often talk about how we would raise our children, and the type of parents we dreamed of being. We wanted our children to fit into our lives, not the other way around. We still wanted to travel, dine out, and have all the same freedoms and luxuries we did before. We'd dream about what our children would look like - hoping they got the best parts from each of us.

Fun fact about me: I'm a planner. I'm getting a little better now that I'm in my 40's. I've come to realise that over planning more often than not, leads to undue stress, disappointment and limits your options. But I still revert to my old ways every now and then.

And back then, I was next level. If something didn't go according to how I mapped it out my mind, I would lose my shit and go into meltdown.

Children were a major part of our plan - actually, they were the centre of it, and we couldn't wait to get started. We were all set and ready to go. So, two years after our first date, we were married in Fiji, in front of our close friends and family. It was magical. Everything was falling into place, just how I'd dreamed.

And that's when the real planning started.

When we got married, I was 33, so we didn't have any time to waste. By then I'd been taking contraception for 15 years, so going off it was a huge deal. When we were on our honeymoon, I stopped taking it. I didn't want to do it sooner because there would be nothing worse than being pregnant while on holidays – right? The irony is thick!

The first morning I left the pill in its packet, I felt like I was free-falling. I loved the excitement and anticipation that just that simple act evoked. But even back then, there was a little bit of doubt that crept in. What if this didn't work? What if I couldn't fall pregnant? After being on the pill for so long, I didn't even know what my cycle looked like. I usually just kept taking the pill each month to skip my period without any thought of the impact it might be having on my body. I still to this day have no idea whether that played a part in our struggles.

At the time, both Craig and I had great jobs that afforded us a very nice lifestyle. But we worked hard. Craig was a sales manager in the tourism industry, and by that stage I was an associate director at my firm in the city.

My job was extremely stressful and time-consuming. As a chartered accountant, I had worked my ass off to get where I was. The harder I worked, the higher I was promoted. The downside was the hours. If there was a project with a deadline, you'd make it work. There were some nights I'd be in the office until 2 am, catch a taxi home, and then head back in at 8 am that day. I was tired, and I was stressed.

In between all of this, we were trying to have a baby.

At first, it was exciting. I had spent my whole life trying NOT to fall pregnant, so I was a bit of a novice, as I'm sure most people are. I had a lot to learn about cycles, ovulation and timing. So, I bought a diary and started tracking. A quick google search told me that ovulation is around day 14, so when it was time, we had sex. Simple, right?

It didn't happen the first month, but that was ok. I comforted myself with the knowledge that I had been on the pill since I was a teenager, so it may take a little time to work its way out of my system. But I was a bit worried. This was my very first taste of the fertility roller coaster - the anticipation of pregnancy, the planning for it, and then it not happening.

It didn't happen the second month either. Or the next. I wasn't used to failure. At school and university, I never failed an exam. Never. And here I was month after month, receiving a big fat negative every time I took a pregnancy test. By then, I'd convinced myself that something was wrong.

Craig and I spoke about the fact that it wasn't happening as quickly as we'd thought, but we never discussed our fears. At the time, we were both scared that we were personally responsible for the negative pregnancy tests each month. What if I couldn't give him the children he wanted? What if he was the reason I would never be a mother?

Our impatience just a few months in sounds ludicrous now, but at the time we were used to getting what we wanted by trying harder. So, we increased the effort.

I started tracking my cycle with a vengeance. This was completely new territory for me. Previously, when my period came, it came. I didn't think anything of it. I googled what the average cycle was and tried to fit mine into it. But it didn't work. I was all over the place

– from 26 days to 35 days. I couldn't work it out. And if I couldn't work it out, how would I know when to have sex? So, I started stressing about it. I started obsessing over it. When I thought it was my ovulation window, we had sex. Not because we wanted to, but because we wanted to have a baby.

It was around this time that Craig started resisting. Maybe it was my desperation, my bossiness or the pressure I was putting on each time – this could be THE one, so it had to be amazing. I blame my addiction to romantic comedies and romance novels for the picture I had in my head of conception. You never see or hear of lovers fighting over when and how to have sex, do you? But here we were, struggling over sex.

I was working hard and doing everything I could to ensure we would fall pregnant. All Craig had to do was provide me with his sperm. All I was asking him to do was have sex with me. A wife, asking her husband for sex. I figured this would be any man's dream. Men think about sex on average 20 times a day, and here I was giving him an opportunity for sex on tap, so why wouldn't he do it?

That played right into my insecurities of being rejected and betrayed in my previous relationship. Perhaps he was cheating on me? Maybe he didn't desire me anymore? I was completely overthinking EVERYTHING.

The truth was that he didn't like being told when and how to have sex. It felt like a chore - like being told to take out the trash. He was feeling frustrated that it wasn't happening either and resented the fact that sex was never in the moment or spontaneous anymore. He never told me at the time, but he was also worried that his sperm wasn't working. Pressure on top of pressure.

Of course, I had no idea what was going on inside his head at the time. All I knew was that he was pissing me off.

Here I was, with my plan in place. At that stage of my career, I was working in our infrastructure team, delivering projects for the government. At the beginning of every project, we would develop a detailed plan of the scope, deliverables and timeframes that would present the correct results. During the day, I had a project plan I was working toward. At night, I was lost.

Not only that, but the organisation I was working for had a paid maternity leave plan, and I wanted to take advantage of it. I could hear my biological clock ticking every single month, and with every negative pregnancy test, it got louder. Looking back, I was only 33 years old, but everything I'd read told me I was already past my prime.

After six months of struggling, with our sex life in tatters, our stress levels now at a record high, we walked into our Doctor's office. He suggested we see a fertility specialist.

Her name was Eva.

She asked the typical questions and did all the necessary tests. It was nerve-wracking, to say the least. Neither of us wanted to be the weak link in this equation. The tests revealed that Craig's sperm count was a little low or as was written on the test results "sub-optimum level". At the time, we joked about them butting heads and not asking for directions - such a typical male trait.

Even though we tried to make light of it, I knew Craig must have been hurting. He was not only surprised at the result, but he was gutted. All the men in his family were baby-makers. His grandparents, his uncles, even his younger sister had two children by this stage. But not him. This was just one more thing that added to his self-doubt.

To be honest, I felt a little relief at the result. Eva indicated that it wasn't such a big deal and that we could just go down the path of IVF. It meant that there was nothing that would prevent us from having a baby. So, the plan changed a little. We could still have our three children from two pregnancies. It just looked a little different. I could do IVF, for sure, right?

We were still in the game, and so began our roller coaster IVF journey.

I must admit, the prospect of starting assisted fertility treatment was a little overwhelming at first. There was so much information, so much documentation, different options, types of cycles. You could do a fresh transfer, frozen transfer, IUI, IVF, ICSI, and there were so many acronyms that you needed a glossary just to interpret.

I'm not a keen researcher so I didn't look into it too deeply, and was led by our doctor on what she thought was best. That was my attitude toward the whole process, really. Perhaps it was a little denial. I was just doing what I had to do – what they told me to do. I knew the result. I wanted a baby. If they had told me to take a special pill, walk backward, hop on one foot, eat kale for a month, whatever – I would have done it. I was very solution-driven. I had a problem, and I wanted it fixed. Now. They were the professionals, so I followed what they recommended.

Looking back, I think that's why I can't remember a lot about our journey. I didn't delve into it, I just did what they told me, and I kept on going. I was focused on the future, not the present moment because there were too many unanswered questions.

If you had asked me to think about how I FELT about all of this, I would have told you to bugger off or that I didn't have time. If you had told me to stop and breathe, and just take stock of where I was at, I wouldn't have because I was scared of what I would find. I didn't want to acknowledge the fears that were staring me in the face. I was so hell-bent on making this happen that I pushed through. I wanted a solution. Feelings and my mental state had nothing to do with it, right?

I couldn't see the roller coaster in front of me – and, how could I? I wasn't prioritising my mental health or my physical health, because I thought this would all be over soon enough. I figured I could deal with it later.

Little did I know, the emotional scars would accumulate over time, and that they would be so deep and so lasting. If I had known that, I would have done things a little differently. I wouldn't have glossed over them. Because the habits I formed over the next seven years, I'm only just breaking down now.

Our first IVF cycle commenced just two months shy of our first wedding anniversary.

Another thing you should know about me is that I'm terrified of needles.

Looking back, I can pin it down to two events that occurred in my childhood.

#1. At school, they would occasionally administer vaccinations. It was like a cattle call. You would line up, lift the arm of your t-shirt, and they would brand you. On one particular occasion, I got myself so worked up, that I passed out. They had to call my mum to have her collect me. It was mortifying. From then on, we went to the doctor to get my needles instead of risking public humiliation.

#2. When I was 10 years old, I contracted glandular fever. I was really sick and had to have weekly blood tests for months. It was horrible. I had a significant amount of time off school, and my skinny arms were so battered and bruised, that it looked like I was a drug addict.

Those two events caused a complete aversion to needles. Still to this day, I can't look at a needle being given regardless of whether it's being administered to me, someone else or even on television.

Needless to say, when they told me that IVF involved receiving daily injections, I was a little nervous. When they said to me that I would have to administer them myself, and into my stomach, I was terrified.

I remember our appointment with the nurse and her showing Craig and I how to do it. I felt sick. Craig said he'd do it for me, but after I saw his reaction when the nurse demonstrated the first injection on me, I changed my mind. I was just going to have to suck it up and get over my fear.

This is a true sign that if you want something badly enough, you will get over your fears and just do what it takes.

To be honest, it wasn't the actual giving or receiving of the needles; it was the thought. I worked myself up about it, but after the first couple of times, it became second nature. Don't get me wrong, I hated it, but it was all part of the process.

At the time I was going through all of this, Craig was preparing to provide his first sperm specimen. I didn't realise, but he was having a lot of anxiety about the process too. He knew his sperm wasn't ideal, and it just played into his insecurities. It felt like nothing came easy to him, he was never enough, and this was yet another speed bump when his friends were procreating quite easily. But we made light of it, and he never mentioned how he was feeling to me.

His first sperm specimen caused quite a few giggles at the clinic. We arrived early on the day in question and completed all the paperwork for the deed to happen. The "specimen collection room" was on the next floor up, so before being ushered into the lift, the nurse handed him the key to one of the rooms. Attached to the key was a large cd case. My mind went wild, imagining what sort of cheesy films were inside there. My thoughts then went to the magazines, the plastic on the couches and those that went before him. I have no idea whether the picture in my head resembled the reality, but that's what I imagined given the assembly line of men waiting to make their "contribution".

Craig being new to the whole sperm sample process looked blankly at the cd case and said to the nurse "Don't worry, I'm not going to steal the keys". He mistakenly thought the large attachment was to deter people from putting the keys in their pocket and not returning them to the front desk. Like in a restaurant, where the toilet door key usually has a big wooden spoon attached.

The nurse and I looked blankly at each other, not sure if he was joking or not. I must have looked a little worried because as the lift doors closed, she leaned down to me and whispered: "He'll work it out once he gets in the room". We both burst out laughing despite the awkward situation. I thought, *Christ, I hope so!!*

We only got halfway through this cycle before Eva realised, I wasn't developing a lining on my uterus. That meant there was no chance for an embryo transfer because it would have nothing to stick to.

I should warn you now - I will not be using the "proper" medical terminology throughout this story. This is my dumbed-down interpretation, and uneducated understanding of what the doctors were telling me was going on inside my body. If you are a doctor and you are reading this, I apologise.

I must admit, that news was a bit of a blow. Up until then, I thought it was Craig that was letting the team down. But now, it was me too. We were both reproductively challenged.

As women, we put so much pressure on our bodies to look and behave a certain way. We are the nurturers, the carers; our breasts are for nourishing our children, our hips are for birthing them, our monthly cycle is for reproduction. Our body is designed to grow a child and mine was broken. I felt a little less like a woman and a tremendous amount of responsibility for our current situation.

I was disappointed in the unfairness of it all, and I was frustrated with myself. I'm a good person. Sure, I have my faults, but everyone does. I was the good daughter, the loyal friend, the dedicated employee. I worked hard, and I had done everything I was supposed to. I ticked all the boxes, so why was this happening to me?

Then the questions started. Did I do something to break my body? Was it because I was on the pill for too long and kept skipping my period because it was an inconvenience? Did I drink too much alcohol, smoke too many cigarettes, or have too many one-night stands in my single days? Did I wait too long to have a baby? Was it my diet? Or my skincare products?

And then it got a little deeper. Is this because I'm not meant to become a mum? Am I being punished for something I've done? Is this a sign I'll be a terrible mum?

The questions were whispers, to begin with. Then they became a little louder. And later they became the white noise that sat in the back of my mind playing on auto-repeat for many years to come.

So here we were, facing yet another roadblock in my carefully laid out plan. Not only that, but there was no tablet I could take to fix it. No injection, no procedure, nothing.

But we kept pushing on with the cycle – Eva told us we would try to get as many embryo's as possible, have them frozen, and work the rest out later.

When I went for my egg retrieval operation, I had no idea what to expect. It was my first time. We walked into the waiting area and I couldn't believe my eyes. There, sitting in a chair in the corner of the room, reading a magazine, was a woman that I worked closely with every single day. I had hidden this entire journey from the people I worked with because I was trying to separate my two worlds. I was also embarrassed, and I didn't want any unsolicited advice. And here it was, my secret double life completely exposed. It was pretty hard not to acknowledge each other, given the fact that we were the only two people in the waiting room. And awkward? Holy crap!

So, we exchanged stories. She was here donating eggs for a friend who was struggling to conceive - an amazingly heroic act. And I was here because we couldn't do this by ourselves. I begged her not to tell anyone at work, knowing that it would probably get back to them eventually.

After that small hiccup, we ended up finishing the cycle with eight eggs, of which five fertilised to become embryos. Five little embryos on ice.

So, what next? How were we going to fix my body so I could use these embryos to make an actual baby?

We had now embarked on our exploration and testing phase, with me being the test subject of course.

Chapter 3

WHAT'S WRONG WITH ME?

This was the beginning of being poked, prodded and considered a "case" instead of a person. We became the patients that doctors debated over in their forums and the topic of discussion in expert panel meetings.

Eva prescribed a cocktail of drugs, the names of which escape me, and a list of instructions to try and thicken the lining on my uterus. It was overwhelming, not to mention that I had no idea what I was pumping into my body. At that point, however, I didn't care, because I was desperate for a solution. After a whole month of sneaking away from work on my lunch break, walking up the hill in my high heels to her small, outdated office to undergo weekly vaginal scans that stripped away my dignity, we were still no further ahead.

My uterine lining was still unresponsive.

What came next was a little more invasive. A Hysteroscopy and Dilatation & Curettage (D & C), which involves a surgical procedure in a day theatre under anaesthetic. Basically, she was going to insert a camera inside my uterus to see what was going on in there and also scrape away what little there was of my endometrium (or uterine lining). It sounds simple, right?

The procedure lasts around 15 - 30 minutes, but it's the lead-up and recovery that takes the time and toll not only on your body, but your emotions. Because I wasn't telling anyone at work what I was going through, I had to make up an excuse. I can't recall which one I used on this particular occasion. However, there were a few standard ones that I accumulated over the years, i.e. I'm going away for a couple of days, I have my mum visiting, I'm not feeling well, I'm going in for a medical procedure etc. Whatever it was, I set my plan in motion to have two days off work - the day of the operation, and a day for recovery.

I was sitting in the hospital admission room, waiting to be wheeled in to learn my fate. Given patience is not my strongest quality, the silence and anticipation were agonising. It was like sitting outside the principal's office to find out your punishment after misbehaving at school. I was conflicted between praying for them to find something wrong with me, and not wanting them to find anything. I needed a reason why my lining wasn't thickening and a cure, but I didn't want it to be anything too bad, like cancer. The Big C diagnosis was always in the back of my mind given I had a history of abnormalities in pap smears, plus the fact that I'd had a surgical procedure to treat a high-grade cervical abnormality previously.

On top of that, it was my vagina we were talking about. It's not like I was going to get my toe operated on. This was a part of my womanhood. Something private, that was going to be on display to a whole operating theatre of people. Not to mention the anticipation of pain afterwards.

After the operation, I woke up in recovery alone, feeling groggy and tender. The nurses gave me some painkillers for the discomfort and told me that Eva would stop by shortly to provide me with the results. The answer to the question - *why is my lining not growing, and is something preventing it?* When she came to see me, I was dozing in and out of consciousness. I knew I wasn't fully comprehending or absorbing much of what she was telling me. Still, the general diagnosis was that they didn't find anything wrong, and we would have to wait for the pathology results to come back on the scraping they took. More waiting!

When Craig came to collect me later that evening after being discharged, I gingerly shuffled out of the hospital, feeling a little fragile both physically and emotionally.

The pathology results did not provide any further clarification or answers for us. Sitting across from Eva in her office when she told us the prognosis, I merely nodded and pushed down my disappointment. So, what was next? She was the expert, so there had to be a plan

B, right? Or had we just executed her plan B? How about plan C then?

It's not great when you're asking the supposed expert the next steps, and they shrug their shoulders. She was perplexed and clearly out of her depth. After sitting there for several seconds looking at each other, she told me she'd speak to a few "experts" she knew. A panel of doctors met once a month, so she was going to discuss our case with them.

I waited to hear back from Eva for several weeks. I tried to be patient; however, we were waiting to find out our fate. Our happily ever after was riding on the solutions that were discussed by these experts. But I gave her the benefit of the doubt. Perhaps the panel hasn't met yet? After a month passed with no word, my heart sunk. I felt defeated. Eva never called us back. Seriously. We never heard from her again. Our first doctor gave up on us and moved on.

Sure, I could have called her. But if I'm brutally honest here, I was scared to call her because I was terrified that the panel wouldn't have any answers either. And for me, not knowing was better than knowing that there was no way forward. That I would never become a mum.

She abandoned us, and that hurt. I may have just been a patient or a number to her, but this was our life. I may have only been a case or a statistic or an unsolved mystery, but to me, this was our future. And it was being ripped out from underneath us.

My heart hardened a little after that, and my anger turned into determination. It never crossed my mind that this was the end of the road for us. This wasn't over by any stretch of the imagination. And if Eva wouldn't help us, I'd find the answers myself.

Something I've come to learn about myself throughout this journey is that I'm driven by the need to succeed. I was hell-bent on proving that the last 12 months of struggles, surgeries, tears and money were not wasted. I was terrified of failing. At that stage, failure looked like selling our white picket family house and saying goodbye to our happily ever after. It was never becoming a mother and never experiencing what it was like to hold a baby of my very own in my arms.

But if you tell me I can't do something, then I will do anything to prove you wrong. I'm motivated by it. Just like the time I jumped out of an aeroplane. It was my 30th birthday, and one of my girlfriends put out the challenge. Would I be prepared to skydive for the big milestone? In my head, I thought NOPE, but what came out of my mouth was a very confident, SURE THING!! I don't think any of my girlfriends believed I would do it. But I went through with it, regardless.

There are a lot of things about our fertility journey that I wish I had done differently, but the one thing that I am SO proud of is the fact that we didn't give up. On reflection, I don't recall any point where I sat back and thought, "I'm done here; I think I'll walk away from my dream of becoming a mum." This journey has taught me

to keep pursuing my dreams and purpose, regardless of what that pesky voice of self-doubt in my head is telling me. After being pushed way beyond the edge of my emotional pain barrier, I'm confident that if I want something, I'm capable of moving mountains to get there. And if I think I can't go any further, I can.......
and I will.

To this day, Craig believes that if he had married anyone else who had faced the challenges and roadblocks we had, he never would have become a father. My determination and drive are what got us to the end. Any normal person would have given up a lot sooner. It was nice to hear, given the fact that he has never complimented my stubbornness before.

Don't get me wrong; there were some days when it felt like the prize at the end was getting further and further away. When it felt like the goalposts were getting moved continuously. Like Mother's Day. It was like being stabbed in the heart. While everyone around us was celebrating, we felt a gaping hole. So, for Mother's Day that year, we decided, along with a few of our friends, to participate in a walk to support and remember those touched by breast cancer. It was a lovely day, and a great way to distract me from my lack of motherhood. But the gravity of what we were going through really hit me. It pissed me off that it was taking so long. I was frustrated that this was happening to me.

But after every setback, we dusted ourselves off, got back up and asked: "what's the next step?"

If a door closed, we searched for a window.

I knew stress affected fertility, so I did my best to reduce it as much as possible. But between the long hours at work, the pressure I put on myself to keep getting promoted, and our fertility struggles, I was at breaking point. I wanted to stay at my high-paying corporate job long enough to take advantage of that very generous maternity leave plan. But the longer this journey took, the more I realised that I had to choose – a baby, or a career with benefits.

So, I made the ultimate sacrifice and started looking for a job with less stress. At the time, Craig was working in the sales department at the iconic Australia Zoo, and there was a job going as a financial accountant in their finance department. I knew I was overqualified, and it was a significant pay decrease. However, I was so dedicated to having a baby and creating the perfect environment to bring a child into this world, that it didn't matter. I applied for the job.

Two weeks later they called me to tell me that, yes, I was overqualified. But they had another role in mind. Their organisation had suffered as a result of the global financial crisis, the downturn in tourism, a killer wet season, and of course the passing of the late great, Steve Irwin. They asked me to come on board to help them restructure and get them back on track, with the promise of becoming the chief financial officer after 12 months. In the back of my mind, I knew it was not the stress-free job I was looking for - it was a huge role. But it was a challenge, and I couldn't resist the temptation. It was a new goal, something exciting, and I knew it would distract me and provide me with a little respite from what was going on inside my head. So, I accepted.

In the meantime, we searched high and low for the magic potion, the magic pill, the magic exercise that would cure our infertility. We googled and received a lot of unsolicited advice from well-meaning friends and family. There was always a story of some fictional person - a friend of a friend of a cousin of an uncle who had found a miracle cure. You know, the fertility tea that Karen drank after she couldn't fall pregnant and now, she has 10 children? Or the unicorn root that Mary took, and she fell pregnant with twins straight away? We were so desperate we gave anything a go.

One afternoon, we were randomly driving down a street when we saw a sign for Homeopathy - a form of alternative medicine using natural ingredients to heal your body. Usually, this wouldn't have gotten our attention, but what caught our eye was the fact that the sign advertised a guarantee for pregnancy – or your money back. Well, sign me up! So, we thought – why not? We had nothing to lose.

We met a lovely lady called Evelin, who, over the next six months, provided us with a variety of drops and pills. She gave us a raft of instructions – what to do, what not to do. We were given ovulation strips and told to have sex on certain days. The pills were specific – no storing near a microwave, mobile phone or hot temperatures. 30 minutes between each medicine. We went on the candida diet, which I must admit, resulted in weight loss for both of us. We were dedicated to the process and followed all the rules.

On reflection, I had gone into this whole exercise with scepticism. Deep down, I didn't believe that this would work. And as predicted, at the end of those six months, Evelin apologised, gave us our money back and sent us on our way. Oddly enough, I had a little bit of satisfaction, knowing that I was right. The money-back-guarantee was a trigger for me. It was almost like I wanted to prove her wrong.

These were the toughest times for me. Sure, it didn't cost us any money in the end, but that wasn't the issue. We had money. I saw it as another six months down the drain. Another six months of watching others fall pregnant around us and leaving us behind. Another six months that my eggs were withering away. And another six months of hoping and praying, all for nothing. We were no further ahead, and I was getting sick of waiting. There was a hole in my faith, in my life and my heart that I convinced myself, could only be filled with a baby. And each month that passed, that hole got bigger and bigger.

Craig, who is not the most patient person in the world, was facing his own fears at the same time. He has a close group of friends from school, and as they were falling pregnant around us, he realised that he was drifting apart from them. The conversations were changing, and he was scared that eventually, we would have nothing in common.

I was so used to being in control. I was kicking goals in my new role at Australia Zoo. Developing project plans and financial models and presenting to banking executives and top-level management. They listened to my advice and took my suggestions on board. During the day, I knew exactly what I had to do to get results. But then I would come home and go around and around in circles. There was no next step, no plan, and I had no idea what to do next. All we had was a dream to have a baby and no one to help us achieve it. We were living in a constant state of hopelessness.

So, we floated for a while.

During that time, we watched others around us fall pregnant and faked excitement for them.

We attended children's birthday parties for our friends and pretended to be having fun.

We watched stories on the news about people abandoning and abusing their children and yelled at the injustice of it all.

When people asked us when we were going to start having children of our own, we told them "oh, when we're ready", and died a little bit inside.

It wasn't fair. But we didn't say anything. We just smiled and pushed it down.

A couple of months later, a girlfriend of mine who was having fertility issues of her own mentioned a fertility specialist she was going to see. She highly recommended him. When I heard his name, I thought this was a sign.

I LOVE signs from the universe. For example, when we first walked through our white picket fence house, we fell in love with it. But what pushed me over the edge was when I walked out the back yard and saw the most beautiful garden of lavender. It reminded me of my nanna, and I figured it was a sign that she was watching over me and telling me to buy it. So that decided it for me.

Crazy? Maybe.

So, this doctor's last name was Wynn-Williams, and my nanna's name was Winifred (Wyn for short), and my dad's middle name was William. It was a stretch, I know. But I was desperate for some indication that we weren't blindly stumbling in the dark. I needed to know that this was part of a bigger plan - that we were being guided. Because right now all I felt was lonely and lost.

So I started searching for meaning. I started overthinking. I started overcomplicating. My mind kicked up a gear in order to cling to some sort of blind faith and hope that this could be it for us.

I found myself, once again, retracting into my unhealthy thoughts. I isolated myself from others as a form of self-protection. Every time someone tried to provide me with advice or a comforting word, it had the opposite effect. A well-meaning comment could trigger my insecurities and bitterness, with my frustration directed toward them. And don't get me started on the insensitive comments. People who complained about how much they hated morning sickness or how much their children annoyed them. It was like a twist of the knife that was already wedged firmly in my back.

I was protecting those around me from what was going on inside my head too. I didn't want them to worry about my mental state. I also tried to protect them from my reactions to their comments, which were becoming harder and harder to push down and ignore. They didn't understand what I was going through, and I didn't want to alienate them or become that girl who always talked about her fertility issues all the time. I didn't want people to perceive me as weak or whining, and I didn't want anyone feeling sorry for me. It was consuming every thought, and I was sick of talking about it. So, I distanced myself.

We pulled back from social occasions and even shopping centres because we would see pregnant women and babies everywhere. Every vision was a reminder of what we longed for and did not have. We were living in this category all by ourselves. We weren't at the singles table, nor were we in the married with kids' group, we were in the married but longing for children category. Basically limbo, with no way forward and no way back to where we had started. A place where no-one wants to be.

On the outside, I was still the sparkly, happy, energetic Jen, but on the inside, my mind was having a field day with everything that was going on.

I would read into everything and have so many horrible thoughts. Thoughts that I never shared with anyone (well, up until now) for fear that they would think I was crazy, or would seriously start worrying about me. I also began to judge others and wondered what made them worthy of becoming parents and not us.

Two months after Craig and I were married and started trying for our baby, my sister had her third child. She had accidentally fallen pregnant. It was at this time in our story, when we were floating, that Craig and I travelled back home to spend Christmas with my family and attend my new little nephew's christening.

This was the point where things were starting to change for us. I felt awkward being around babies because it was this love-hate push-pull effect. Don't get me wrong, I loved being around babies, but it hurt because it was a reminder of what I didn't have and longed for. I was self-conscious around them - it felt like everyone was watching and waiting for our reaction to having children around us, and talking behind our backs. They weren't, but I was paranoid.

Mason was a little blue-eyed, blond-haired, pale-skinned cherub. He looked completely different from my sister's previous two children, who were dead wringers of her and her husband - dark chocolate eyes, brown hair and tanned skin. They joked that Mason was supposed to be mine, given the fact that I too have blond hair, blue eyes and pale skin. Everyone thought that the stork had put the baby in the wrong basket/person. I laughed, but it hurt.

It also got my overactive mind thinking. What if that was right? What if he was our one chance, and now it was gone? Now, writing it, it sounds like the most ridiculous thing. So absurd that it may not even make it through the editor's review, and form part of this story. But at the time, these are the conclusions that my crazy mind was drawing. Because I was utterly lost, I would search for signs. But I would completely overthink them, and come to the wrong conclusion. I would give something meaning when it didn't even warrant acknowledgement.

Walking into Dr Wynn-Williams office for our initial consultation, I felt hopeful for the first time in a long while. The reception area was classy and spacious with a coffee machine in the middle, filtered water jugs and vases of fresh flowers. Quite the opposite compared to Eva's cramped treatment room. In our appointment, we relayed our story from beginning to end. He listened and assured us that this wasn't the end for us yet. He gave us options, and exactly what I was craving. A plan of attack, which included different drugs, protocols and treatments we could use until we found something that worked. It was a huge weight lifted from my shoulders - instant relief.

So, we began yet another process of me being poked, prodded and treated like a human guinea pig.

Over the next four months, I was pumped full of different drugs to try to stimulate the growth of my endometrium. We began where we left off with Eva and started on high doses of oestrogen tablets, then moved to hormone injections to prepare my uterus to transfer one of our frozen embryos. I prayed that my body had magically cured itself. But at every scan, despite the numerous blood tests showing normal hormone levels, my endometrium did not budge or grow.

After that, we moved to high levels of vitamin A tablets, aspirin, even higher doses of oestrogen and even viagra (yep!!) pessaries to increase the blood flow to my uterus. Well, apparently that's what we did. This has all been pieced together from my medical records because, at the time, it was so overwhelming that I didn't know whether I was coming or going. My emotional state was fragile, to say the least. But I pushed it down, and a numbness took over. And that became my new norm.

There was only one constant throughout the whole process. At every scan, it was the same result. Endometrium is unresponsive.

The final step was exploratory surgery once again. There were a couple of adhesions found during my last hysteroscopy, so they wanted to rule out Asherman's syndrome - which is a uterine condition, characterised by the formation of adhesions (scar tissue) inside the uterus and/or the cervix. So, they booked me in for another hysteroscopy. I was getting good at this by now. I was completely detached from my body and was just following instructions. Take this, do that.

Once again, I went through the same emotional build up as my previous surgery with Eva. I made all the necessary preparations. I took two days off work, creating some kind of excuse as to why I wouldn't be in. I stocked up at home with a heat pad, painkillers for any cramping afterwards, plenty of books to read, movies to watch and comfort food. The surgery was planned in a different hospital to my previous one, so it was like starting from scratch again. A different doctor and unfamiliar surroundings. They told me to refrain from eating and drinking for eight hours before the operation. I had completed the necessary consent forms, had my gown, booties, cap and blood pressure stockings on. And I was laying on the gurney waiting for them to wheel me into surgery. I could do this.

The anticipation and fear at that moment made me tense and frightfully cold. You know there are risks in every operation, especially when an anaesthetic is involved. And I was always conscious of the dangers around it, given my mum had a history of reacting badly to the drugs. They usually had a hard time waking her up, given her low blood pressure, and when they did wake her up, she was violently ill. So, there I was, all alone at the end of a strange hospital corridor, trying to be brave and calm myself down before being wheeled in to find out my fate yet again.

After what seemed like forever, Dr Wynn-Williams walked in and apologised. There had been a mix-up with some paperwork, and the hospital wasn't allowing him to perform the surgery today. I could tell he was furious and embarrassed.

I couldn't fathom what I had done to deserve this. It was like I was being punished all over again. I wasn't sure how much more of this I could take. I tried to make him feel better by saying it was ok. But it wasn't. This wasn't ok. I wasn't ok.

I slid off the gurney, took my surgery outfit off, pulled my clothes back on and called Craig to come and collect me. I walked out of that hospital feeling more defeated than ever.

And then we had to do it all over again. A new hospital, a new time and a new roller coaster of emotions. Luckily that operation went through without a hitch. In fact, I was the first operation of the day and was wheeled in without having to wait. I appreciated the effort, and couldn't help thinking that he felt sorry for me and was showing me a little mercy.

When he called a couple of days later with the results, I was nervous. I wanted something to be wrong, but I hoped it wasn't anything too serious. But alas, I passed with a clean bill of health. No answers and no solution. And just like that, we were at the end. Again. The doctors were perplexed. There was nothing medical or scientific they could find that was stopping my lining from growing. They had tried all the treatments in journals, consulted other specialists they knew, and they all scratched their heads in wonder.

My freaking body just wasn't responding. My body was betraying me. And there was no one else to blame or point the finger at. This situation was no one else's fault, but my own.

To cope with all of the ups and downs throughout this phase, we travelled. That year we made our way through Europe and the Middle East - Santorini, Athens, Prague, Abu Dhabi and Dubai, as well as a driving holiday around Tasmania. Don't get me wrong; it was amazing. But we were trying to fill the hole that a baby had made in our life - it was our consolation prize.

Sometimes I think not knowing why was the most frustrating. At least if there is a diagnosis, there is a reason, and perhaps a treatment. But there was no physical or medical reason for why my body wasn't working.

It sounds bizarre that you want something to be wrong with you. You would choose something to be wrong, so you know, rather than being healthy with no explanation. We just wanted an answer to our question.

It was at this point that Dr Wynn-Williams sat us down and told us that our chances of ever conceiving naturally were slim to none, and that our best chance of having a baby of our own would be via surrogacy. We could use our embryo, but we would have to implant it in someone else. This meant that instead of me carrying our baby, feeling it grow and getting to know it before it was born, someone else would get that honour. I was devastated.

And it made me bloody uncomfortable given my control-freak tendencies. I like doing things my way; I'm not that great at delegating because let's be honest, no one can do as good a job as me. And here I was having to outsource the one job I had been dreaming about my whole life. Release control and become a passenger in our quest for a child. It was SO wrong.

I was numb.

I had a clear picture in my head of my pregnant body. Have you ever watched the movie Notting Hill, with Julia Roberts who plays a glamourous and successful movie star and Hugh Grant who is an awkward book store owner? It's the perfect romantic fairy-tale of how two people randomly come together and live happily ever after. My favourite!! The final scene in the movie is where Julia Roberts and Hugh Grant are relaxing in a large public garden. People are practising Tai Chi, children are running around laughing and playing, and families are picnicking in the park. The camera zooms in from behind to show Hugh (or William Thacker) sitting on a park bench reading a book, and Julia (or Anna Scott) laying across the seat with her head resting on his lap, and her eyes closed. They are holding hands, and as the camera zooms in, you can see her hand resting softly on her bulging pregnant belly. It was such a beautiful moment and one that I had been secretly longing for myself.

But I wasn't going to have that moment anymore. I had been robbed yet again of the fairy-tale.

The practical side of me pushed those feelings down even further and put a lid on them. I'd deal with them later.

What's next?

And in walked our Angel.........

Chapter 4

HEARTBREAK AND HOPE: OUR SURROGACY ROLLER COASTER

O ur Angel was Renee - my sister in law.

She had seen us struggling for two years and witnessed first-hand the heartbreak that we endured month after month.

To be honest with you, I can't even remember how the conversation went. I do know that we didn't have to ask. She offered. It took me by surprise that someone would volunteer their uterus and nine months of their life so automatically and freely. And I think I was shocked because we didn't have an extremely close relationship. Don't get me wrong, we got along fine, but it's not like we were catching up regularly or sharing our deepest darkest secrets. And this was such a huge deal. Craig and I weren't sure what to make of it. When she first threw the flippant comment out there months before it became our only hope, I think we all laughed. It wasn't serious.

But now it was. On the drive home from our doctor's appointment that sealed our fate, we made the phone call to Renee. You'd think that a conversation that started with "were you serious about having a baby for us?" would deserve a face to face catch-up over a nice dinner, but we needed an answer. We were sitting in limbo, and she was our last hope. So, there we were, sitting in our car with Renee on speakerphone, asking if she'd have a baby for us.

Her response? Absolutely!! But she had to speak to her husband Nathan first.

It sparked something in me.........it was a new plan. And it was hope, even if it was just a glimmer.

Could this be real? What would this mean? What was the next step?

I think we were so hell-bent on pushing forward with this path that we ignored the risks involved.

Today, on reflection, I can see that it was fraught with danger.

What if something horrible happened and it broke up the family? What if something didn't happen, and Renee had to live with the guilt of not being able to give us a child?

What if it dragged on too long and was too tough, and we ended up resenting each other?

We were naive and had a perfect picture in our head of how it would unfold. We'd transfer our frozen embryo, she'd fall pregnant, and nine months later we'd have our baby. Renee adored being pregnant. She'd told me she never felt healthier, more energised, or more beautiful than when she was carrying her babies. And falling pregnant was something that came easy to her. She had been on the pill when she fell pregnant with her first son and fell pregnant again within weeks of saying it was time to give her son a sibling.

Of course, I had never been pregnant before, so I had no idea the impact that it has on a woman both physically and mentally. And it was the one thing that I craved the most - I saw it as a huge privilege, so I figured we were doing her a favour. We would all benefit. As a result, we ignored the questions that were in the back of our minds and pushed them aside. We didn't want to know.

When Craig's parents started voicing their doubts, we thought it was because they were traditionalists. We thought they were worried about what other people would think. So, we pushed their concerns aside too.

Looking back now, with a completely different mindset, I realise those doubts came from a place of love and genuine concern for all of our emotional wellbeing.

Renee and Nathan had two boys of their own who were five and nine at the time. How would we explain this situation to them, and would they be able to handle it?

When Nathan, Renee's husband started resisting, we thought it was because he was selfish. I'm deeply ashamed of believing that now, given the fact that he is one of the most caring and selfless people I have ever met. Nathan was desperate for more children, but Renee was vocal in her stance that their family was complete. It was a very sensitive issue, and we never found out the impact that it had on their relationship until I began writing this book. For that, I am truly sorry.

The truth is, we didn't explore the reasons for everyone's apprehension surrounding our surrogacy arrangement, because we didn't want to know the answer. We were scared of what it would mean.

All we saw was a story we made up in our head. That we had finally found a way to have a baby, and they didn't want us to. They weren't happy for us. They wanted us to stop.

This is the point where it is apparent to me that we were completely consumed in our fertility journey. Of course, we were oblivious at the time, but looking back now, this is where we started to lose sight of logic and reason.

From my experience, there are a series of stages that you go through. I'll coin it the "Fertility Consumption Lifecycle" for these purposes.

When you start down the path of trying to conceive, you experience excitement at the thought of adding a baby to your family. You have your job, your friends and your hobbies that form your life – and then a desire for a baby is added to the side.

Then when it doesn't happen, it takes over a little more of your thoughts. If you choose alternative methods to conceive, like IVF or use natural remedies like acupuncture, it takes over a little more of your time (and your finances) too.

After a little while longer, it takes over more of your thoughts and becomes more than just a desire. It becomes an obsession. You see babies everywhere – in your favourite television show, in magazines, on the side of a bus, billboards, at the park, in your shopping centre, down the street – EVERYWHERE!

Instead of your job being a method of earning income, it becomes an escape from the constant thoughts and a way to afford your next fertility treatment. So, you throw yourself into work. Your hobbies are replaced by researching the magic cure for infertility. Your time with friends is spent talking about where you're at with baby-making, and your friends' circle splits between those who do have children and those who don't. You gravitate toward those who don't have children because you don't want the constant reminder of what you don't have. It's too painful.

And before you know it, it has consumed everything. Your fertility journey and struggles have become your life, and you're sitting to the side wondering why you have this constant deep feeling of sadness, frustration and hopelessness. You don't recognise the person you've become, and you're so used to putting on a front and pushing those feelings deep down inside that it becomes a habit.

Your fertility journey officially consumes you. There is no YOU; you have become the PROCESS.

So that's where we were. After two years of trying to conceive, our fertility journey had finally consumed us.

Looking back now, the concerns that our family were raising were reasonable. But tell that to a bull after waving a red rag in front of his horns. Renee said yes, however, so we were going with that answer.

Then we were referred to a surrogacy specialist, Dr Ben Kroon. He was terrific, and we all loved him. Over the next couple of years, we formed a great relationship with Ben, or as we affectionately referred to him (behind his back) - Kroonie. He didn't beat around the bush, but he genuinely wanted us to have a baby and wanted to see us succeed. You could tell he loved what he did. He went above and beyond for us – from late night and weekend appointments, even when he was supposed to be on holidays. But most of all, we trusted him – to tell us the truth, give us the best advice, and guide us. And when you're on this journey, you need that. Because there is so much happening for you on the emotional side, you're not thinking rationally.

Not only that, but he was a nice guy too. So, we all made a great team. And at times, that's what this felt like. We were a team – he was the coach telling us about the plays and co-ordinating everything, Renee and I were the players passing the ball (or embryo's) to each other, and Craig was the waterboy (he'll love that, I'm sure) providing support and encouragement when we needed it.

Together we tried to make light of situations that were usually stressful and sometimes downright awkward. We joked, laughed, but never cried. I can count on one hand the number of times we cried in front of each other.

I didn't realise it until I started writing this book, but neither my husband, my sister-in-law or I can remember details about our journey. How many cycles we went through, or how many fertilised embryos we had. It was a complete blur.

And it was because we were in survival mode.

For us, it wasn't about the journey; it was about the destination. We put our heads down and were running. We were so desperate to get to the end and get the hell off this vicious roller coaster that we closed off the rest of the world and focused on the prize - that bouncing baby at the end of the tunnel.

Our method of communicating with Renee was usually via text. It made things easier to stay at arm's length. There was less pressure rather than being in each other's faces all the time. We respected each other's personal time to process the hurdles as they came up. And they did.

We weren't present, and we isolated ourselves. We didn't deal with things that were going on, and we didn't talk about it because what we were going through was too hard to comprehend.

I remember at Christmas one year; we'd just done a transfer and were waiting on the test results. The family was all gathered celebrating the festivities. I was nervous to see her because I was afraid that she already knew our fate. When she walked in, I looked at her and she shook her head just a little. At the time, the rest of the family were unaware that we had done a transfer. My heart broke. We didn't talk about it. There were no words spoken. And that was it.

I thought if we didn't talk about it, the feelings and the memories of disappointment would magically disappear once we had our baby. I know for a fact now that this is untrue. While the wounds heal over, the scars of infertility remain for life.

What I didn't know at the time was that we were experiencing grief. I had always thought that grief happened when someone died. So I didn't believe I had a right to claim those emotions. But I did - because I was grieving that picture I had in my head of how my path to motherhood would happen. I was grieving the loss of myself to infertility. Later on, I was grieving lost babies.

And I was trying to come to terms with the fact that bad shit happens to good people.

Writing this book has been the explosion that I have needed. Facing emotions I had pushed down, trauma that was laying low.

In the end, I had to once again refer to our medical records to piece it together, and I was shocked at the number of cycles we went through. Nine in total. Nine times we hopped on that roller coaster. Which meant we failed eight of those times. But after each failure, we picked ourselves back up, dusted ourselves off and carried on. We were so freaking tough. So determined and steadfast in our pursuit. THIS would not break us.

From the outset, surrogacy was an overwhelming process. There are lots of rules, regulations, and steps you need to take to get the legal sign off to proceed.

I resented every step of it. Every hurdle seemed like a slap in the face. Commercial surrogacy isn't legal in Australia either. Which means that if you aren't as lucky as us to have a selfless angel in your life that volunteers, you're screwed. You're forced to go offshore, at the risk of breaking the law. Of course, if you go overseas, the costs go up exponentially, once again limiting the people who can go down that path.

There is no medical subsidy or rebate for surrogacy either which makes the costs compared to IVF, exorbitant. As if the fact that you can't carry your baby isn't punishment enough, our medical system and government treat you like a second-rate citizen too.

Firstly, Ben had to make a submission to a surrogacy committee - he had to state our case proving that this was the only option for us, given my "medical" condition, which was still unknown. If the medical board approved, then we could proceed to the next stage.

We then lawyered up. We engaged a lawyer to draw up a surrogacy agreement. Renee had to hire a separate lawyer to provide her with advice on what she was agreeing to. If I'm honest, the process of drawing up a surrogacy agreement was a little frustrating and utterly redundant. It's not an enforceable contract, so not worth the expensive paper it's written on.

Any baby born via a surrogate in Australia is deemed to be the birth mother's child. So, Renee would legally be our baby's mother and would have all rights, up until we legally adopted. Regardless of the surrogacy agreement drawn up, at any point in time, Renee could have changed her mind and kept our baby.

Of course, that would have made our annual Christmas family get together very awkward. However, it was still a possibility and something that weighed on my mind.

And then there was counselling. We had to undertake a joint session and undertake psychological testing. And it wasn't just Craig and me; it was Renee, Nathan and their children, Bailey and Jai. We had sessions together, separately, in person, over the phone, written tests, you name it. It was intense - especially with children involved - you never know where a conversation is going with a five and a nine-year-old. At the same time, there's that voice in your head, hoping that the questions asked and the answers you provide, don't reveal that you're crazy or too unstable to go through this journey.

In the end, however, we were all deemed to be emotionally stable enough to get through the surrogacy process. The counsellor did up our report and sent it off - Phew! Next hurdle jumped over.

Finally, after almost six months spent jumping through hoops and lodging documents, and copious amounts of money spent on legal fees and counselling, we were given the green light to start our surrogacy cycle.

We honestly thought it was full steam ahead from here on. And it was. We just didn't realise the ride was going to be so bumpy and long.

So here we go. Strap yourself in......

We were all so excited. This was shiny and new for us, and we were all set to make a baby. We had our signed surrogacy agreement, a rubber stamp from the fertility authorities and we were ready.

Our first transfer used one of the embryo's we had frozen from our first IVF cycle. This was excellent news for me. It meant skipping the egg collection process of jabbing myself in the stomach with a needle and filling my body full of hormones for two weeks. It was still nerve-racking though - there was a chance the embryos wouldn't live past the thawing process or grow enough to implant.

It was Craig's job to ring the laboratory each morning to see how our ice babies were travelling. Did they survive the night? Were we still on? I couldn't make the phone call myself. The anticipation was excruciating. Craig didn't mention it at the time; however, if the results from the lab were disappointing, he would sit there contemplating how to break it to me. How would he word it to make the news a little less devastating?

Luckily, one embryo survived. We all breathed a big sigh of relief. I took this as a sign that things were finally going our way. That we had endured the heartache and the hurdles we were meant to face, and now it was over. Transfer day came, and we all presented at the day theatre. My insides were jumping around with anticipation and excitement. This was it. We were going to have a baby and begin our happily ever after. Renee and I put on our medical gowns, caps and shoe protectors and were ready. It was GO time! We were all in good spirits and filled with hope. We took pictures and laughed nervously in the waiting room. We had no idea what to expect beyond the closed hospital theatre doors – this was a first for us.

To be honest, however, I felt a little like a third wheel. I wasn't part of this equation; however, I felt like I needed to keep control of the situation. I felt a little pang of uselessness. They were implanting our baby into someone else. If I'm completely honest (which is the whole point of this book), it hurt a little. But I was so excited that this was happening, so I pushed down that feeling and kept imagining the result. We were making a baby! I should be grateful. So, I planted a fake smile on my face to mask my pain and those horrible thoughts going through my head.

So here we were, in a sterile theatre, Renee with her feet up in stirrups, trying to make light of an extremely tense situation. The call eventually came through from the lab that our magic little embryo was ready to be collected. Ben proceeded to the collection window with an unusually long implement in his hand and came back with our embaby on the end of the stick. I kept thinking – is it really in there? How would they know? Insert more awkward conversation.

I was shaking and tense. I have no idea how Renee was feeling, however, given the fact that she was the one with her legs in stirrups, I'm sure she was more stressed than me. You would never know with the amount of laughter happening, albeit more nervous giggles than anything else.

Everything went smoothly, however, and each of us went back to our respective jobs for the day as if nothing had ever happened. And then there was the dreaded two-week wait. That window of time where you're just waiting, and hoping and praying that the baby gods are smiling down upon you and that your embryo sticks. The two weeks where it feels like time is moving backward, not forward. Where you try to distract yourself but are doing a miserable job. So, we waited. And waited. And waited. In reality, it was only 12 days, but it felt like a lifetime. Then the result……..negative.

FUCK!

We were gutted, but no one said much. We didn't talk about it. I had no idea what Renee was feeling at the time; however, after talking to her now, she had a complete feeling of failure. She felt guilty that we had put our trust in her, and she had failed us, causing us more heartache and money.

From my perspective, I felt guilt. That we were dragging Renee along on this journey with us. Every time she had to take drugs, use what sounded like horrendous, icky pessaries or rearrange her life to attend doctors' appointments, I felt guilty. And now she was experiencing our disappointments too. We were exposing her to our emotional roller coaster, and that wasn't something I'd wish on anyone.

I felt completely powerless. I had no control over what was happening inside Renee's body. I couldn't tell her what to eat or encourage her to reduce stress. I knew first-hand how frustrating it was when people told you what you should be doing. So, I had to trust that she was looking after herself.

Craig was in the middle. Stuck in between two extremely strong-willed and determined women, watching us both suffer. He was discussing things with his sister that no brother should know. The conversations were awkward, to say the least. At the same time, he was acting as a go-between with his parents and sheltering them from the process as much as possible. We didn't want them to worry, so we were only providing snippets of information.

From here on out it became a desperate race. We were all so hell-bent on protecting each other from hurt, feeling guilty and failure, that we went full steam ahead. ALONE.

After the first failure, something inside me died a little. It was HOPE. Up until now, we had never been at the point of testing for a positive result. We went into the first cycle with hope and anticipation, and when it didn't happen, it bloody hurt. So, I associated the pain at the end, with the hope and excitement I had felt at the beginning. I thought if I stopped hoping, then maybe it wouldn't hurt so much when it didn't work out.

I approached every cycle after that with reservation and scepticism. I thought, if this doesn't work, then we can just go around again. Before each cycle had even ended, I was thinking about the next one, and the next one.

No wonder I can't remember the details of what happened on our journey. It was such a heavy burden to carry. I lived through it, but I didn't feel any of it. I was completely numb and emotionally spent.

There is a quote by Lao Tzu that says, *"If you are depressed you are living in the past. If you are anxious you are living in the future. If you are at peace you are living in the present."*

I spent seven years floating from the past to the future. Seven years of depression and anxiety. It came out of me as a whole raft of emotions and reactions. Anger and frustration being the most common.

In a meeting at work one day it was revealed to me (by accident) that my nickname was Cruella de Vil – the villain from 101 Dalmatians. That hurt a lot because I knew I wasn't that person deep down. But of course, they didn't know the struggles I was going through, because I was living a secret double life. Strong and driven on the outside, anxious and depressed on the inside.

On reflection, my choice to live mainly in the future and keep planning for the next cycle was self-preservation. I understand that. But it did more damage to my emotional state than I anticipated. It also started a horrible habit of pushing all my emotions down. A habit that I'm only just beginning to rectify now.

Don't get me wrong; I have fully embraced my story and everything it entails. If I had to choose my path or an easier/smoother/less expensive one, I would still choose mine 100 times over because it had a happy ending. It also taught me a lot of lessons and made me who I am today.

But I wish someone had told me this when I was being consumed. When I was wondering why it wasn't working.

When I was overthinking things, and concluding that this wasn't happening because I wasn't meant to be a mum.

I needed a voice of reason, but because I was internalising, my voice was the only one I was hearing. And that voice was telling me that this wouldn't work, that I didn't deserve to be a mum, that this wasn't meant to be, and that I was a failure.

So, after that first negative pregnancy test, we pushed our emotions down, got back up, dusted ourselves off, and tried again. We still had a couple of embryos frozen, so we decided to use them. Unfortunately, we didn't get to the transfer stage with this round. Each morning Craig rang the laboratory to see the progress of the thaw until they told us that none of them had survived.

FUCK!!!!!

Back to the drawing board. This meant doing the full cycle, including the egg retrieval, and needles in my stomach. Oh, joy. Not only that but as I mentioned before, it was bloody expensive. Each full cycle would cost us around AUD$10,000 a pop. But we hadn't gone this far, to only go this far.

So, we kept pushing forward. For every egg retrieval, I underwent acupuncture treatment to ensure I created the best quality and quantity of eggs possible. It made me feel good to know I was doing everything in my power (physically) to ensure this worked not only for us, but mostly for Renee. I would do this until we succeeded, but I knew there was a limit for Renee.

I hadn't fully thought through the impact that this would have on her body. Every morning she had to insert a progesterone pessary in unimaginable places and take drugs to make sure her body was ready to receive the embryo. Then after the transfer, she would have to do the same. I was conscious that she had signed up to have a baby for us, not ride this roller coaster of drugs and emotions. I felt guilty every time she had to do something invasive. But she was such a trooper.

As our journey progressed, I struggled with a lack of control. I already felt like an outsider, and on more than one occasion, test results were provided to Renee instead of me. She would receive the phone call, and I would find out second hand. I would be waiting on the phone call, trying my best to be patient, only to find out that the receptionist had provided the results to Renee and not me. When I rang up to make specialist appointments, they wouldn't be able to find my file, because it was under Renee's name. It hurt so much that they didn't even know who I was. It felt like I was being squeezed out.

It all came to a head at one of our embryo transfers.

On the morning of the transfer, we were feeling the anticipation and excitement build. On the drive into the hospital, we received a phone call from Renee asking where we were. We got the time wrong. She was about to go in for the procedure, and we were still 15 minutes away. My heart sank, and I started panicking. Craig dropped me off at the front door of the hospital, and I sprinted to the lift pushing the button rapidly. Renee was already in the theatre with her legs up in stirrups. They didn't wait for me. There was a mad dash by the staff to get me into my theatre clothes, so I didn't miss the whole thing. And then it hit me like a tonne of bricks. They didn't need me for this. They were implanting my potential baby into someone else, and I wasn't required. I never felt more like an outsider than at that moment. Despite rushing into the room just before the transfer occurred, it was too late. The damage had already been done to my frail ego.

I feel an intense amount of shame even verbalising this. I feel like an ungrateful teenager. What kind of person feels this emotional about losing control? Who cares who was called? Who cares if I wasn't there? It seems so trivial. It shouldn't matter, but it did. I was already carrying a deep amount of insecurity around not being able to fall pregnant, and it felt like I was becoming redundant in this process.

In the midst of my emotional turmoil, I received a phone call from a close friend of mine. After catching up on what we'd each been up to, there was a pause in the conversation. She said, "Jen, I have some news, and I wanted to tell you before anyone else.......I'm Pregnant. Sorry." I could literally hear ringing in my ears and felt myself spiralling downward. I glanced at the bottle of wine across the kitchen bench and knew where I was headed straight after I hung up the phone. I just had to hold it together and get through this call. So I pushed it down and put on my best "I'm happy for you" voice. I told her it was fantastic news and that I was fine. But I wasn't. Not even close.

I could feel her pity, and it made me feel weak. I tried my best to be happy for her. I did. What kind of person can't be happy for their friend when something good happens to them? I struggled with a tremendous amount of guilt and shame. If I was a better person, surely I wouldn't feel this way. If I was a better person, I'd be able to feel happy for her, and sad for me. But I was just pissed off.

You see, when my friend came to our wedding and celebrated our nuptials with us, she was single. And in the four years we had been struggling to have a baby, she met a guy, was getting married and was now pregnant. It made me so angry. Everyone was moving forward with their lives, but we were in this constant holding pattern. Our friends were celebrating the birth of their second and third children, and we were still on the starting line.

From that day, I started avoiding friends who I thought may tell me they were pregnant. When I'd catch up with them, I'd monitor whether they had a glass of wine. And if they didn't, I'd go down into that dark hole all over again.

It was a long road, and we went through all sorts of cycles. Nine times over. Just writing that makes me feel a little sick. I had no idea how large that number was. I know that sounds silly. But we honestly didn't count.

Some cycles included egg retrieval, embryo transfer, and then a negative result. In some cycles our embryos didn't fertilise, so we didn't get to the transfer stage.

But one particular egg retrieval sticks in my mind. For those of you who aren't familiar with it, egg retrieval is a long, emotional and suspenseful process. It involves two weeks of injecting yourself with high levels of hormones. Daily blood tests, scanning, monitoring and prodding to make sure they time everything perfectly. The doctor counts on the screen how many follicles are present each day, and it becomes a tally. Almost like watching the lotto or a horse race - how many numbers are you going to get, how fast are they growing, how big? The timing was everything.

On the day of your egg retrieval, you go to the hospital and walk into the waiting room. It's filled with other women who are doing the same thing. It's intense. But there is no conversation, and no one is sharing. We all have our protective armour on, our walls up, and are sitting in our thoughts. You sit quietly and wait for your turn. It's like an assembly line, and women get called one by one. You give each other a small smile, silently wishing them luck, knowing you'll see them at the other end. You then get wheeled into the theatre where the anesthesiologist is waiting to put you to sleep.

Looking back, this was my favourite (if I had to choose) part of the whole cycle. I know that sounds weird. You're packed full of eggs (any more and you'd start clucking like a chicken) and feeling a little discomfort. But it was the feeling of going under anaesthetic that I loved. I could finally relax and be at peace. I had done my job and tried my hardest, and now the rest was out of my control. Finally, someone was looking after me. It was in this moment that my mind stopped racing with the possibilities, the gruelling and punishing thoughts, the what if's, and the sadness and anger. In that moment of counting backward from five to one, I was finally free. There was no tossing and turning at night, no bad dreams. It was quiet. And even if it was just for an hour, it was like a little slice of heaven.

It never lasted long enough for me, though. After the procedure, it was back to reality. You wake up in recovery with a number written on your hand. That number represents the number of eggs that were collected. While it may seem impersonal, regardless of what state you're in, as soon as you open your eyes, you need to know the number. Depending on who is still in the recovery room, there is occasionally chatter between the women revealing how many eggs were collected. And usually, one woman is laying silently, crying. Well this day, that woman was me. There was a perfectly formed 0 on my hand.

When Ben came in to see me, I cried in front of him for the first time. Usually, I kept up a pretty brave face, but I didn't have it in me this time. This was raw; I was tired, devastated and frustrated. Zero eggs. It wasn't that they didn't fertilise; it wasn't that the transfer wasn't successful. This was all on me. I had done everything that they told me to do, and yet I had failed……again.

And now we had to start at the beginning all over again.

This part is always quite ironic to me. As women, we go through a whole invasive and painful procedure to extract our eggs. But the men? They get to jack off into a cup while watching porn - quite a broad spectrum in terms of experience. Don't get me wrong; however, it's not all smooth sailing for the guys - they have to put up with our mood swings and watch us suffer helplessly from the side-lines. But if I had to choose, I know who I'd want to be in this scenario.

But we kept going. You may be thinking at this stage - why? Why would you put yourself (and your family) through all of this?

Well, on cycle number six, we were given a glimmer of hope. I remember it well, because the morning of the embryo transfer, we arrived at the clinic. The nurses took Renee's vitals and discovered that she had a temperature. Usually, that wouldn't be cause for concern; however, if her temperature was too high, her body would absorb the embryo, making the whole process a waste. We were all tense and silent. I couldn't believe this was happening. They gave Renee some Panadol, and we went through with the transfer. We weren't hopeful. But low and behold, 12 days later, the test came back positive. Holy crap - we had done it! We made a baby!

The next few weeks were a euphoric blur of dreaming and planning. It was a surreal moment given the fact that in the four years we had been trying, we had never had a positive result. The excitement, anticipation and relief were enormous. We told our family, and they were ecstatic for us. Our little family was finally going to be complete.

Our excitement was short-lived; however - it all came crashing down seven weeks later. In the dingy public toilet at a sports carnival she was attending for work, Renee discovered that she'd started bleeding. She called Craig on the way home to break the news. We were all gutted and in shock. I don't think we'd ever considered that this wasn't going to stick. I guess we figured we'd been through enough, that our happily ever after was long overdue and had finally arrived.

The next morning, we picked Renee up to take her for a scan. She was wearing dark glasses which did little to hide her puffy eyes. I know it sounds ridiculous; however, this is the first time I grasped the emotional and physical impact of our choice to involve Renee. The car ride was tense. No one spoke. I don't think we were capable of it, and I didn't know what to say. We were all pretending that we were ok, and were doing a piss poor job of it.

When we arrived at the clinic, it was sombre greetings from Ben, which was a stark difference to our usual banter and joking. You could have heard a pin drop when the picture came up on the monitor. Not knowing what we were looking for, I knew what we were listening for. That hopeful sound.....gadoonk gadoonk gadoonk gadoonk. That would have been music to our ears, but we never heard that noise. The scan revealed we were no longer pregnant. It was over before it even began.

Like us, Renee was devastated. To make matters worse (as if you needed to), it was her son's 10th birthday. And instead of being able to enjoy the festivities, she spent the night, doped up on painkillers, at the 10-pin bowling birthday party they'd arranged. She had to smile at their guests and help the kids, while making frequent bathroom stops to see our hopes fade away.

What made it a million times harder was the fact that we had done this to her. She was going through one of the most traumatic experiences a woman can endure, and was now a member of a club that no-one wants to be a part of. And this was all our fault.

Miscarriage – the silent struggle that 1 in 4 pregnancies end in. The result that no one talks about. The shame, the guilt, the devastation.

I had no idea what she was going through, which meant I had no idea how to comfort her. Hell, I was still trying to work out how I felt about it and could barely put one foot in front of the other myself. After that, we all retreated to our corners to grieve in our own way.

My girlfriends and I had pre-planned a getaway for my birthday at the time, and it just so happened to be that weekend. I had been given a bottle of expensive champagne and was planning on opening it and announcing to my friends that we were finally pregnant. But instead, it was consumed in between sobs as one of my girlfriends, who knew the grief of miscarriage all too well, consoled me.

I just prayed that Renee was getting support from somewhere too, because we weren't capable of providing it to her.

After that, we decided to take a break.

Renee and her family took a well-earned holiday. For the last four years, Craig and I had planned our life around our fertility journey. That was fine for us; however, I failed to consider that now Renee had put her life on hold too – a life that also included two small boys and a husband. But this latest cycle had proved we all needed to take a step back and regroup.

I'm ashamed to admit this, but in the back of my mind, I was already 10 steps ahead. Would this end everything for us? Would Renee want to try again after this blow? For me, this experience gave me hope. If we got here once, we could do it again. But I was being selfish. I was only thinking about what I wanted, not the impact this would have on everyone around us.

So, Craig and I waited for the verdict. Was Renee in, or had she had enough? We didn't want to push our hopes on her or make her feel guilty. She had to make this decision for herself. But the anticipation was unbearable.

Thankfully Renee felt the same way as us. This had given her hope too. Any other surrogate would have thrown in the towel by now, but not this amazing lady. Call it stupidity or downright stubbornness, but we decided we would see this through to the end. And we weren't done yet.

By this stage, we weren't telling anyone when we were undergoing a cycle. Not even our family. It was too painful for everyone involved. It's hard enough trying to reconcile everything we were going through in our own heads, let alone trying to explain it to someone else. I didn't want anyone's sympathy, and I certainly didn't need them to dramatise events that were happening or get caught up in our roller coaster. It was emotional enough without having to comfort others when there was a dip in the road. And the pity - oh man I was sick of people feeling sorry for me. So, we travelled the remainder of our path alone, with very little support apart from each other.

Now I'd love to say that we were a close-knit team and there for each other - but we were just trying so hard to survive and get through this, that we didn't have room for high fives or words of encouragement. To be honest with you, we didn't share how we were feeling or what we were thinking. I can't speak for Craig and Renee; however, I was scared if I spoke the truth, it would unravel this whole journey.

Surely any sane person would have given up by now.

We did two more negative cycles before receiving a hot tip.

My personal trainer at the time, who was also undertaking IVF, was seeing an acupuncturist who specialised in fertility. Her name was Anne, and she came with an incredible 100% success rate in helping women going through IVF fall pregnant. At this stage, we would have accosted the tooth fairy's assistance if we thought that was going to help.

Renee loved Anne and went every fortnight.

I asked Renee what it was that was so amazing. She said "I would walk into her clinic room and the tears would silently, instantly flow. She would wrap me up in a gentle embrace, help me onto the table and the soft music and smells of her tiny 1st-floor room coaxed out the fortnight's woes. She would calm me, counsel me and treat my physical and emotional ills with tiny flexible needles and a giving soul. I would have the most peaceful, deep, hour's sleep and leave refreshed, blissful, and ready to take on the world."

It sounded amazing, so even if it didn't work, we were grateful that Renee was getting some much-deserved peace on our roller coaster.

It wasn't until I started going to see Anne myself a year later that I grasped the enormity of what Renee was gushing about. Anne was a miracle worker who could get you to relax until you fell asleep, drooling like a baby, and also release all that emotional baggage.

And by that stage, we were all carrying around trunk loads of crap. I remember some days driving to see Anne, only to have tears streaming down my face blocking my view of the road. My body was releasing all its emotional baggage before I had even arrived at my appointment. Poor Anne wore the brunt of both Renee and eventually, my own path to pregnancy.

What Anne provided was a safe space to release the emotional energy trapped inside us. She provided an outlet for us to let go of the pain, stress and anxiety we'd been holding onto that had been suffocating us.

Anne proved to be the release we needed. On our next cycle, we fell pregnant with Luca.

Chapter 5

YOU KNOCKED UP
YOUR SISTER?!

Seven months after our miscarriage, I ran my first ever half marathon. When I say it like that, it gives the impression that there were other running events occurring afterwards, like the second and third time I ran a half marathon. By all means, assume away. The truth is that I've always claimed to dislike running. I loved the thought of it, and I know people rave about how great it is to clear the mind, but I was never a fan. It hurt every part of my body, from my ankles to my knees to my chest to my head. And clearing my mind? The only thoughts that were going through my mind usually related to how much my body hated me. So, it came as a complete shock to me when I made the unexpected decision to run a half marathon.

To be honest with you, I think I was so desperate for a distraction from the fertility roller coaster we were on, that when a girlfriend suggested it to me; I said yes. Here was a prime opportunity to get fit AND immerse myself in something that had nothing to do with sticking needles in my stomach and getting my vagina examined. Sign me up!

So, I started training. Slowly. Bit by bit. I was terrible - but I had a plan. And if you give me a step by step guide on what I have to do, and when I have to do it, I'll get it done. I had a training schedule, and I stuck to it. I hated every moment apart from the euphoria and satisfaction that came at the end of a run. But I must admit, I had never felt so strong both physically and mentally as I did at that point in my life. I was making progress, slowly but surely.

After eight cycles, five egg retrievals and a miscarriage, we were all at breaking point. So, for me, training for a half marathon was the distraction I needed. It provided me with something else to reach for aside from motherhood because, for the last four years, my only goal had been to have a baby. This journey had consumed me from the inside out. It left me wondering who I was and what my life was about, apart from conceiving. It had become an obsession.

Running was the distraction I needed to disperse the fog I'd been living under. It got me through that last cycle without having a major meltdown, and for that, I will be eternally grateful.

For Renee, it was her appointments with Anne.

During my training, we received our very long-awaited, much-anticipated news.

We were pregnant again!!

It was one of those moments where you weren't sure whether to celebrate or not. On the inside, I was doing a major happy dance, but on the outside, I was terrified. Or vice versa. Whichever way it was, the point is - we never got too excited. But it was so hard not to.

During this journey, you learn how to temper your emotions for self-preservation reasons. It was a tense wait until our scan day. We picked up every phone call from Renee with trepidation. Would today be the day our world crumbled again? We didn't tell anyone we were pregnant this time. We just couldn't take the chance.

Finally, it was time for our appointment with Ben. We were all trying to play it cool, but I knew if Craig and Renee were feeling half the anticipation and excitement that I was feeling, they were doing an excellent job of hiding it too. Renee was up on the table, and there was complete silence as we looked at the big screen. It felt like a lifetime before Ben hooked up the machine and put that wand under the sheets. And then we heard a very welcome sound.....gadoonk gadoonk gadoonk gadoonk.......a fast thumping that had us all squealing for joy. Renee had tears streaming down her face, and even Ben let out a whoop. We had reached our first hurdle, and it felt like a huge weight had lifted from our shoulders. This was the beginning. We still had a long way to go before we could truly celebrate, however, this was the closest we'd gotten to something we'd been fighting for, for over four years.

The next two months moved at a snail's pace. We were waiting to tell everyone. And of course, no one suspected a thing. One of the benefits of using a surrogate is the fact that you can hide it. I wasn't running to the bathroom with morning sickness, no sneaking crackers under my desk at work, and no sign of a baby bump. Plus - one of the BIG bonuses - I could still have a cheeky glass of wine!! It was a perfect plan to throw everyone off the scent.

The day finally arrived for the long-awaited, much anticipated 12-week scan. This was the big hurdle for us. Come to think of it; they were all big hurdles. We knew if everything looked good here, we could finally get excited and share the long-awaited news that we were expecting, with our family and friends. Before we met Renee at the clinic, Craig and I stopped to get some lunch. I remember ordering and putting food in my mouth, but I didn't taste it. Butterflies filled my stomach along with a feeling I can only describe as masked hope. Where you feel hopeful, but you're trying to push it down and not get too excited. Not open up your heart fully to the possibility that this could be it.

At the clinic, we tried to lighten the mood by cracking jokes and making small talk. But that wait before our scan was excruciating. On the other side of this appointment, we would be either excited or devastated. When they called Renee's name, we all piled into the room. The clinician looked at us oddly. Why were there three of us? And why was Renee's brother in the room? Awkward! So, we explained our story......yet again. It was met with surprise and a gentle nod of understanding. Then the clinician went to work moving the equipment over Renee's stomach, taking measurements and snapping pictures. All the while we were glued to the screen looking and waiting. We had no idea what we were looking at, but we were all waiting for confirmation that everything looked normal.

It wasn't until she looked at us and asked whether we wanted to know the sex of the baby that it started to dawn. If there was something wrong, she wouldn't be concerned with asking us this question. Of course we wanted to know! We were always going to find out - I needed to plan the colour scheme for the nursery, clothing styles, bedding type, narrow down our baby name list, the lot. So, this was a bonus for us. Not that it mattered either way at this stage - we weren't fussy. A living, breathing and healthy baby was just fine.

It's a boy! She exclaimed. Not only could we (kind of) see actual arms, legs and other body parts, but we were having a baby boy. Shit just got real. This wasn't an egg; it wasn't an embryo; it wasn't a positive test; it was a baby boy. And he was ours!

At that moment, we let our guard down a little and felt pure excitement and joy.

I remember calling our parents from the parking lot of the radiology clinic to tell them. It was the most incredible feeling. We had done it, and we could share it with those that had followed and supported us throughout our journey. There were tears. But this time they were tears of joy.

The next few months were surreal. We were having a baby, but for all intents and purposes, there was no evidence. Sometimes I had to pinch myself. We had to keep reminding ourselves. There was no morning sickness, no blood tests, no changes in my body. On the whole, it was wonderful.

But there was also an element of fear involved. Renee was spending the first nine months of our baby's life with him 24/7. I wasn't. He would be born and not know our voices. He would be more familiar with Bailey and Jai, his cousins, than he would with us. We would be strangers to him. What if I couldn't calm him and the only person who could was Renee? I would be mortified.

Being a first-time mum is hard enough to wrap your head around. You read a million books on how to feed them, put them to sleep, bath them, you name it – and I was reading them all. But there was nothing on how to deal with the emotions or fears I was experiencing. How do you get past the fear that your baby will love his Aunty more than his biological mother?

And every now and then, I had a pang of sadness. I didn't get to feel our little boy kick from the inside, I couldn't feel him growing, and I couldn't talk to him and read him bedtime stories.

But I pushed those feelings deep down inside because if I voiced them, it would make me ungrateful. I know better than anyone else who suffers from infertility, the struggle to create a happy and healthy baby. This was indeed a miracle, and here I had it but was still a little disappointed. If my pre-pregnancy self could manifest herself from the past to the present, she would punch me in the ovaries for even thinking that. But I'm not going to sugar coat this for you or me. I'll say it out loud........*I wished things were different. I wished I was carrying my own baby.*

Renee felt guilty for robbing us of our pregnancy experience - when she went to the doctors and heard our little boy's heartbeat and we weren't there, she felt terrible. Now, how amazing is this woman? She was carrying a baby for us - growing an actual human inside her body for us. She had endured a miscarriage, countless transfers, not to mention progesterone pessaries up her woo hoo. And SHE felt guilty for getting to know our baby before we did?

Of course, I told her to stop being so silly. We were there for all the significant moments, so it was fine.

In reality, however, and in the back of my mind, I was still a little disappointed that I wasn't able to feel the kicks and talk to my little boy. This is NOT how I had imagined my pregnancy.

This is one of the themes that kept on coming up while I was writing this book. Nothing went according to the way I had imagined.

The plan. The picture. And that's what kept knocking me on my ass.

Life doesn't always go according to plan. But what if our plan limits us? What if it keeps us small?

If you'll indulge me just a moment while I digress, to demonstrate my point.

Two years beforehand (after our second failed transfer), Craig and I travelled to the United States and Canada for a holiday. We had friends who were getting married in Toronto, so we decided to build our dream holiday around it. We flew into San Francisco and drove to Banff, Lake Louise. It was October, so it was getting a little bit chilly, and the mountains looked majestic with snow-capped peaks. We were staying at The Fairmont, Chateau Lake Louise, which was right on the lake and as we were driving up, it started lightly snowing. When we awoke the next morning, it was like a fairy-tale, our very own winter wonderland.

After Lake Louise, we were off to Las Vegas. With every wedding, there must be a bachelor party, and no bachelor party would be complete without the obligatory trip to Sin City. Vegas never seems to disappoint. I'd been there before, and it always sucks you into the hype and excitement with lights, entertainment and excess in every way. We stayed on the strip in a fancy hotel and while Craig did the things you do at a bachelor party (casino, strip club, shooting hall, cocktails in ridiculously tall glasses), I explored the strip.

From there it was off to LA where we did all the touristy things you can think of - trekked the Hollywood walk of fame, visited the wax museum, caught an LA Lakers game, toured Warner Brothers Studio where we formed part of the studio audience of the Conan O'Brien Show, and went on a tour of celebrities houses. A tour of people's homes seemed so cool at the time, and we had a hoot, however, when looking back through my photos now, it's a bunch of pictures of people's houses, and I have no clue who they belong to. Plus, it all seems quite stalkerish to be honest. My dream of running into Chris Hemsworth and us bonding over our Australian accents and love of Byron Bay did not come to fruition, unfortunately.

Then we were off to Toronto for the wedding. While we were there, we made the one-hour drive to Niagara Falls, which was amazing; however, it was such a cold, and wet day, it was a little miserable. It rained the whole time we were in Toronto, but the wedding was brilliant, and that is why we were there.

The plan was to go to New York next, followed by Orlando, and then Hawaii on the way home.

New York was MY part of the trip. Craig could have Vegas if I could have New York. I have always dreamed of going there. It has always been on the very tippy-top of my list of places I wanted to visit, given my obsession with Sex and the City. Plus, every romantic film gets shot in Central Park. I was super excited.

We were so caught up in holiday mode however, that we didn't pay attention to any of the weather warnings. We had no idea that there was a hurricane about to ruin our holiday. On the day we were supposed to fly into my dream destination, Hurricane Sandy hit New York. It flooded the streets, tunnels and subway lines. It cut power in and around the city and according to wikipedia, did $65 billion worth of damage. We were so desperate to get there despite all flights into the area being cancelled, we considered hiring a car, catching a bus, just so we could catch a glimpse of the Big Apple.

In the end, we admitted defeat. We went straight to Orlando and spent an extra three days there. Craig, who is an avid theme park fan, was more than a little thrilled. I, however, was bitterly disappointed. I was supposed to be on top of the Empire State Building and running through Central Park, not meeting Mickey Mouse and hearing *It's a Small World* over and over again. I know that sounds a little ungrateful - oh boo hoo, you didn't get to go to New York, so you had to endure Orlando and experience Disney World instead. Yes, I agree. But it wasn't according to my plan, and I didn't live out one of my dreams.

It was not how I'd pictured it.

Which brings me back to our pregnancy.

When I'd pictured having a baby, it was always with me being pregnant. I mean, of course it was - I'm kind of stating the obvious here. In my perfect pregnancy movie, I had the cutest baby bump (all belly of course, not an inch of fat). I had cravings of peanut butter, pickles and ice cream (without the calories or fear of getting gestational diabetes). I would spend hours rubbing my bulging belly, talking to my baby bump, feeling him/her kick and dreaming of the things we'd do together.

This was a little different; however, I ignored it. We decided to make the best of a situation that wasn't exactly ideal. Because it wasn't me that was pregnant, we were able to go on an epic babymoon.

You guessed it - when Renee was six months pregnant, Craig and I flew to New York!!! And this time we planned a trip where New York was the main destination. It wasn't a measly three days squeezed in between Toronto and Orlando. Our holiday was ALL about New York. We spent almost a week exploring every single amazing sight.

We walked along the Hudson River where Sully miraculously landed that plane, jogged through Central Park, soaked up the excitement and the bright lights of Times Square, walked the Highline, and ate pizza in Little Italy. We took a million pictures of squirrels, went to Fifth Avenue and shopped at Tiffany & Co and FAO Schwartz. Experienced Grand Central Station (shake shack!!!!), watched the Lion King on Broadway, went over to Brooklyn and walked across the Brooklyn Bridge, shed a tear at Ground Zero, went to Wall Street and the New York Stock Exchange. We caught a ferry to the Statue of Liberty, saw Derek Jeter hit a home run at Yankee Stadium, kissed on top of the Empire State Building. Recited lines from Ghostbusters in the New York Public Library, took a helicopter ride across New York, had an ice-cream sundae at Serendipity and rode in a horse and carriage through Central Park. We finished off our holiday with a few nights at Manhattan Beach in San Francisco.

It was hands down the best holiday ever! It surpassed all of my expectations. Looking back to our original holiday plans two years earlier, I can't imagine squeezing all we did into three days. If we had gone to New York back then, it wouldn't have been the same. And we probably wouldn't have gone back a second time either.

So, while I was disappointed that Hurricane Sandy ruined our first trip to New York and that our holiday didn't go according to plan, it ended up being a good thing. At the time, we couldn't see it through our disappointment. But looking back now, I can see that we were supposed to go back and do it properly. And we did.

This taught me that when things don't go according to plan or the picture I have in my head, it may be because there's another, much better plan around the corner.

And there were a lot of moments on this journey when I thought; this is not how I pictured it. Probably none more so than the day I found myself on the train to work, with a cup of sperm nestled safely in my handbag.

How? It was simple. During one of our IVF cycles, Craig had to provide a fresh sperm sample to the clinic.

His place of employment was nowhere near the IVF clinic; however, I worked down the road from it. So, we decided that I would make the delivery and then head off to work.

For those of you who aren't aware, there is a time limit between ejaculating (sorry) and deposit, so the clock was ticking. That morning I waited (not so) patiently for him to do his thing, begging him to hurry because I was going to be late for the train. Once the deed was done, I swiftly took said sample and after checking the lid was secure (several times), put it in my handbag and hopped on the train.

Ensuring my handbag was warm under my arm (another requirement for the sample), the other passengers sitting next to me on the train were completely unaware of what they were in close proximity of.

At the time it seemed quite normal, which was an excellent indication that my version of normal was off the charts, bat shit crazy.

But here I was, far beyond that picture in my head.

Trying to rationalise and come to terms with the path we were going down in our heads was one thing, explaining it to others was a whole different ball game.

Because the surrogacy law at the time was relatively new in our state, people weren't familiar with the concept. We were among the first to test the legislation that was in place – we were guinea pigs. When we told people our story, it was either met with two reactions.

It either made people cry at how touching our story was and how heroic and selfless Renee was, or it caused confusion.

We didn't see the irony of our situation until we explained it to some of Craig's mates. "What, you knocked up your sister?!" was exclaimed in horror. Perhaps we didn't explain it well enough. Or maybe their mind was wandering somewhere it shouldn't be. Either way, it became the running joke.

Craig and I were out to dinner at our local restaurant one Friday night having pizza and wine. We were excitedly going through our baby name list. We'd narrowed it down to about 10 names by this stage and were debating each of them in detail. How did the name sound with our surname, and were there any rude combinations that he'd get teased about later in life? The couple next to us overheard our conversation when we mentioned a name that just so happened to be the same as their little boys. We started telling them that we were trying to narrow down our baby names. I saw their eyes move to my belly and the glass of wine in my hand. We quickly explained our situation and they congratulated us.

We started looking at child care centres for when I would eventually go back to work after being on maternity leave. Most of the good centres are tough to get into with long waiting lists, so we didn't want to miss the boat - plus my planning instinct kicked into high gear. If I couldn't do anything else to help grow this baby, I'd make sure we were super-prepared when he eventually arrived. Our walk through child care centres was sometimes a little awkward. They usually looked at me like I was crazy. We always had to explain that, yes, we were almost due to have a baby, but no, I wasn't pregnant. Either that or I was hiding it remarkably well. It was usually met with a nonchalant nod, which I think was just an un-comprehension of our story.

When it came to prenatal classes, we booked a private lesson to avoid confusion. We didn't need to know about how to birth a baby or how to breastfeed. All we needed to know was how to keep our baby alive once the stork delivered him.

My work was great about the whole situation. In reality, I could have waited a lot longer to tell them about my pregnancy. I wasn't showing, and I wasn't sick. But I was so nervous about breaking the news. It was the first time I had to explain what was happening to people who had no idea of the struggles we'd been going through. No-one at work knew about the epic fertility journey we had been on. It was just such a private thing, and I didn't feel it was a topic that needed to be discussed in the lunchroom. Plus, if I'm completely honest, a part of me was still ashamed about the path we'd had to take to get here. It was never a short - "guess what? we're pregnant!" Cue hugs and squeals of joy and questions about how you're feeling etc. It was more like a "so we've been trying to get pregnant for the last five years, and then we couldn't, so we used a surrogate, and now we're pregnant." Pause for awkward silence, and questions - lots of questions. With answers that still hurt to tell.

I remember the day I finally told my boss we were pregnant, so clearly. My voice was quivering, my hands were shaking, and I cried. It was such a surreal moment. It was a moment I had played over and over in my mind for five years, and here I was, finally breaking the news.

When Craig told his work, it was a little different. For those he was close to, he divulged our full story, but with the others, he merely let them assume our path was quite regular and that I was pregnant. There was no need to share something so personal to everyone.

The people at my work who heard about our story congratulated us. There were quite a few that had missed the news and were completely oblivious, however. Why would they suspect any different? I certainly didn't look pregnant.

At my farewell party from work, it was.........well, it was just plain weird. There were nappy cakes, bags with baby clothes and other gifts. It looked like your regular farewell for the lady going to have a baby, minus the lady carrying the baby, of course. There were, however, a few people that asked me where I was going. The look of disbelief when they found out I was going on maternity leave was priceless. This was not conventional by any stretch of the imagination.

And of course, I could work right up until the baby came too. We were booked into the hospital for a caesarean section because Renee has a cone-shaped uterus and can't birth normally. Yes - every part of this conception, from beginning to end was scheduled. So, my final day at work was Friday, and our little boy would be arriving the Wednesday after.

We did have an extra thing on our to-do list before our baby arrived. Tell the neighbours. None of them knew the private struggles that we had been going through the last five years, and why would we share that with them? It was a personal journey and not one that you talk about over the fence when you're pulling the garbage bins inside on a Friday afternoon. It occurred to us that if we mysteriously brought home a baby, they may call the police. So it was the weirdest conversation ever and went something like this...........''Hi neighbour, just wanted to let you know that we're having a baby in a couple of days, and we didn't want you to think that we'd stolen him, so we thought we'd better tell you now. No, I'm not pregnant, but Craig's sister is having a baby for us. No, it's entirely our baby - my egg (cringe) and Craig's sperm (double cringe). But the doctors told us that there was a low probability of me falling pregnant, so we went down this path.'' Yep, pretty awkward. I have no idea what they thought, but I'm sure it was the topic of conversation at their dinner table that night.

Because Renee lived an hour away from us, and we were having our baby at a hospital further down the road from her, we booked into an apartment for a little mini-break before our baby boy arrived. I remember the moment we closed the door and left our house for the last time as a family of two. Knowing the next time we re-entered those doors, we would have a newborn baby in our arms was exhilarating yet terrifying. My heart was seriously about to burst with excitement. There was so much anticipation. This baby was five years in the making, and he was only three sleeps away.

Chapter 6

LUCA: THE MUCH ANTICIPATED AND CELEBRATED ARRIVAL

We spent the next couple of days relaxing as best we could. Our friends with children had told us to dine out and go to the movies as much as possible beforehand, so we were trying to savour every moment. I remember our last dinner, and our last full night's sleep (albeit a little interrupted by the excitement).

That morning I woke early with butterflies in my stomach. I'd packed a bag with clothes for myself and our baby. One of the main reasons we had chosen this particular hospital was because it would allow me to stay as well. They acknowledged that our situation was a little different, that we were all playing a part in this pregnancy, and they accommodated us.

Ordinarily, it's just the mother who stays in the hospital room and spends the first few nights with her baby. And of course, in the eyes of the law, I wasn't the mother of our baby.....Renee was.

Over five years I had pushed my body to its limits by injecting high levels of hormones, almost double-digit anaesthetics and operating procedures, an emotional roller coaster filled with trauma, and invested copious amounts of money in our quest. And here I was, an outsider, asking permission to be involved. It was just one more little blow to my already damaged ego.

We also had to get permission for the three of us to be in the operating theatre. Usually, it's only two people allowed, i.e. the mother and a support person. Of course, Craig and I both wanted to be there, so when we explained our situation, we were thrilled that they granted us special permission.

We met Renee at the hospital. We were all excited - us for our new arrival, and Renee to get her body back. This baby had taken its toll on her health - she'd had kidney infections during the pregnancy and had been on medication to get her through. Add to that the poking and prodding endured not only during the nine months prior, but also the two years before that on our IVF journey. She was looking forward to a well-deserved beer too!

Unbeknownst to us, she had written a journal of her pregnancy to give our baby. It was a beautiful dedication to him and contained pictures of her growing baby bump, tales of the adventures he'd had albeit on the inside, and told him how much he was loved.

While we waited for the various tests and monitoring to occur before they wheeled us into the operating theatre, she handed the book over to us to pass on to our little boy. I was able to experience and understand her side of the pregnancy. To say I sobbed like a baby is an understatement. Even now, after rereading the journal, it still has the power to bring me to tears. But today they are different tears. When I read it for the first time in that hospital room, they were tears of relief, a little sadness, and the emotion of the enormous changes that were about to occur in our lives. We had all been through so much to get here. To be honest, I was a blubbering mess. But today when I read it, they are tears of gratitude and so much joy, it feels like my heart is about to explode.

I'm going to share with you the first entry and the last one before our little boy came into this world -

We finally got to see you today! The REAL you! Not just a tiny circle like we saw five weeks ago.

You are an amazing medical miracle that your mum and dad have been working so hard to make a reality for so many years.

After so much heartache they agreed to let you grow in my tummy.

I can't imagine how hard it is for them to not experience, every day, what I get to see and feel.

They have had to forfeit one of life's most incredible experiences and entrust their most prized possession to me until you take your first breath.

I hope you can fathom how much you are adored!

You gave us quite a surprise today when we heard you are a boy! For years we have all been certain that when you arrived you would be wrapped up in pink, the first of many things you are going to do that amaze us!

As I hopped in my car to head home from your scan, I heard your mum and dad let out a hilarious excited giggle! They are so excited and can't wait to hold you!

Only 28 weeks to go........

Yes, she is one amazing lady. Are you crying yet? No? Well, wait until you read this entry....

It's 3 am on your birthday.

We finally get to meet you today! I'm already tearing up.......it's going to be an emotional day, but in less than 12 hours, you'll be in your parent's arms finally.

I'm going to miss the little nudges you always give me, and my new built-in table to sit my plate on.

Your mum and dad are so excited! And nervous, but mostly excited.

I'm so grateful they let me grow you. You feel like a victory for me. An achievement. Something I've done that I can be proud of.

I can't wait to watch you grow and learn. To see the sheer joy you give your parents, just by being with them.

I hope you always remember how incredible you are. How adored you are. No matter what happens in your life, you'll always know how badly you were wanted in this world and how incredibly ecstatic we are to have you here.

Happy Birthday xoxo

Our baby really was loved. We had loved the idea of him for five years already. This experience brought us all so much closer than we were before. It was like we were the three musketeers, fighting against all the obstacles put in our path. Ok, maybe not the three musketeers, but we definitely felt stronger together than before. It was a sense of pride. We had fought so hard to get here, and we did it. It was a feeling of great accomplishment.

His cousins had formed a cute bond before he had even come into this world too. They had spent the last nine months with him - they had watched in wonder as he had grown and moved inside their mum's tummy, felt his kicks, and had spoken to him daily.

So back to the hospital. I'll be honest with you - I was bloody nervous. I had no idea what to expect from here. When the midwife had come to our house for our private prenatal class, she taught us how to wrap, feed, change, and keep a baby alive. But birth? Well, there was no need. We were having a stork delivery. So, you'll understand now that I had NO idea what was going to happen next. I hadn't watched any of those horrific videos of babies being born in a frenzy of afterbirth, screams and blood. In fact, I had done everything in my power to avoid it. It just wasn't my thing and a completely unnecessary piece of viewing given our circumstances.

The closest I had come to witness a birth was when my sister sent me some photos of my niece after she'd been born. It was all beautiful until a picture of my niece being pulled out of her stomach covered in all sorts of gunk surfaced. I promptly told her it was downright offensive and to keep that sort of stuff tucked away in her private album in future.

Maybe I should have paid a little more attention? Now I was entirely out of my depth. All I knew was that we would go into the operating theatre where they would cut our baby out, clean him up and hand him to us. I didn't worry about the logistics up until this morning.

It was at this point that time seemed to be going backward. We just wanted to get this show on the road. Nurses would come in to monitor different things, take measurements and write them all down on a chart. I felt a little like a third wheel. Each would assume that this was Renee's baby (well, why would you believe any differently?) and must have wondered why her brother and sister in law were in the room, in addition to her husband. If they looked at us a little weird, we explained it.

After what seemed like an eternity, the time finally arrived. Our whole party headed to the operating theatre. My body was tense, I felt a fake/nervous smile cramping my cheeks, and my hands were shaking. This was it! The moment we had been planning for was finally here. We all got dressed in our theatre outfits - hair hats/shower caps, booties for our shoes and face masks. We looked like we were ready to walk into an episode of ER. I wouldn't have minded seeing George Clooney at this stage - he sure would have broken up the nerves I was feeling. Man, I must have gone to the bathroom a million times that morning!

The moment they gave Renee the epidural I started to cry. It was such a build-up. I had held so much in up to this point, and it was such an emotional time. Of course, I tried to wipe away the tears quickly. When they put the needle in her spine, I looked at her face (because there was no way I was looking at that big ass needle going in) and she scrunched it up in pain. I felt this intense wave of guilt. She was going through physical pain for us - her stomach was going to be cut open, and she was going to have additional scars, just for us. Guilt. Gratitude. Overwhelm. How would we ever thank her for this?

And then we all made our way into the operating theatre filled with a team of doctors, nurses and students. We had cameras, video cameras, the lot. This was the most loved and anticipated baby, and we were going to catch every single moment on camera. And we did.

Both Craig and I sat at Renee's head (because there was no chance I would risk fainting and missing this moment for the world - plus the alternative would be just weird) and tried to comfort her as best we could. I think we were cracking horrible jokes, just trying to lighten the mood. It was SO intense.

And then our baby boy arrived. There was a flurry of excitement, lots of scurrying around and then silence. I'm sure it only lasted a couple of seconds, but for us, it was a lifetime. And then there was a cry. Luca had entered the world. And exhale.

Once they cleaned him, we gathered around the incubator trying to catch a glimpse of our little boy. I remember having this intense feeling of accomplishment and relief. We had done it.

Craig had his arm wrapped around me as we watched the doctors monitoring and doing all the checks to make sure our little boy was perfect. Of course he was. He leaned over to whisper something in my ear – I figured it was going to be something amazing, words of wisdom, something touching. "He's got massive balls!". Yep. What a way to break the tension. He had a point though - they were enormous. We then entered into a conversation with the nurses about our tiny baby's big balls.

When they finally placed him in my arms, it was miraculous. I couldn't believe this was happening. I felt an intense amount of love, and I never wanted to let him go. We brought him over to meet his Aunty Renee, who was watching on with pride.

After that, they whisked Renee away to recovery, where her husband Nathan was waiting for her. Craig and I made our way back to the hospital room with our baby and started our bonding. We both did skin to skin contact with him to try to ease both of our anxiety. It was such an amazing feeling. The next 24 hours were a whirlwind of learning how to feed a baby, bath a baby, and introducing him to our family.

That first night was a shock, though. I went from having a full night's sleep every single night to waking up every 30 minutes. Typically, you'd ease into the world of interrupted sleep by having a baby kicking inside you or pushing on your bladder to force you to go to the toilet. But not me - it was cold turkey, and it was a shock.

By morning I was exhausted. I felt so bad every time Luca woke up because Renee would wake up too. She had already done so much for us - she deserved a good night's sleep. I could tell she was exhausted too. When Craig came in the next day with coffee and hash browns, I almost leapt on him. Is this what motherhood felt like? Constant exhaustion? I think more than anything else it was the emotional exhaustion. We had just gone through a massive change. Life was normal one day and completely thrown on its head the next. I know that happens to everyone; however, it was seriously like a stalk had just delivered a baby to us.

Don't get me wrong - I was in tip-top shape physically (remember I'd run a half marathon just eight months beforehand), but I was worn out emotionally. But I pushed it all down and ignored it once again.

When Nathan arrived that morning, he looked exhausted too. Amid our euphoria the day before, his father had passed away. He had been diagnosed with terminal cancer around the time we'd fallen pregnant with Luca. Nathan was holding it together, but just barely. Now he had to break the news to Renee, who was already in a fragile state, having just given birth to a baby that brought with it all the usual emotional ups and downs.

I never realised until writing this book how much Nathan had also endured for us. For the last two years, he was dealing with the fact that his chance to have a third child was coming to us, and now he was grieving for his father in amongst our joy. His strength and positivity were unbelievable, super human-like even. I know he was crumbling inside because I knew exactly how it felt to lose your father to cancer. Losing a parent is like losing a piece of you, so my heart went out to him.

Craig and I wheeled Luca in his capsule down to the waiting room to give Nathan some privacy to break the devastating news to Renee. When she found out, of course, all she wanted to do was be with Nathan. And here she was stuck in a hospital bed having just undergone childbirth and a major operation that comes with a caesarean. But like the Angel she is, she switched from helping us bring a child into this world, to grieving an amazing father in law and supporting her husband while he came to terms with a world without his father in it.

And that is what led a woman who had given birth via caesarean section just 24 hours beforehand, checking herself out of the hospital and moving on to save the next person.

Looking back, I wonder whether the grief associated with the loss of her father in law distracted her from the fact that she had just given birth to a baby she'd carried inside her for nine months, and then handed him over. I wonder how she would have felt if things didn't go down the way they did. Would she have felt the emotional let-down that comes after childbirth? Would she have felt sadness or loss at no longer carrying our baby?

Since then, I've spoken to Renee about whether she feels a deeper connection with Luca. The answer is yes; she feels a need to protect him fiercely and ensure he is happy. Is it any different to how an Aunty feels about any other nephew? Yes. But the most apparent emotion is a sense of pride and accomplishment. That we achieved and created something great. That we got back up and kept fighting for him.

Over the last couple of months, I've heard stories from other women who have also been surrogates. While they felt a deep connection with the baby they carried, they all emphasise that at no point did they feel stress or sadness in handing the child over to its intended parents.

I don't know why, but that surprised me. Maybe I've been watching too many movies where it doesn't end well. But it just doesn't seem to be a big deal. You go into it knowing that it isn't your baby, so you don't get emotionally attached.

Take my work colleague who was donating eggs for her friend, that I bumped into in the fertility clinic all those years ago. It resulted in twins, so now she is the biological mother of two children belonging to someone else. When I asked her if she felt an emotional attachment to them, she said no. Sure, they were her eggs, but they weren't her children.

Up until now, it had been a fear of mine. What if Renee didn't want to hand over our baby? What if she had grown so attached that she couldn't do it? Looking back, the number of fears I had was innumerable. But most of them were irrational, and things I had made up in my head. I was giving them meaning and wasting my energy, giving them power when they didn't deserve any more than a shrug.

"My life has been filled with terrible misfortunes, most of which never happened." ~ Mark Twain.

Yep, I hear you, Mark. Fears keep you small, and I was small for a long time.

Before Renee left the hospital that day, there were a few technicalities and complications we had to deal with. Given I wasn't Luca's mother in the eyes of the law, I also wasn't the patient they had on record. But I wasn't comfortable going home with a baby just yet. We'd only just learnt how to bath him, and he still had some tests they had to run. The hospital was amazing, though - they permitted me to stay with Luca as long as Renee signed him over to us.

In the lead up to that second night in hospital, I was feeling a little apprehensive. Renee had been my safety net on the first night. While she was there, the handover wasn't complete, but with her gone, it was all on me. The night before had rattled me a little too – this was tougher than I thought it would be, and now it would just be Luca and I. But that's the way it goes, isn't it? Things are usually tougher than you expect them to me. But I survived. In fact, it was much less stressful. We'd introduced a pacifier, and I didn't have to worry about waking anyone else up.

The next day when Craig arrived, I was ready to go home. It was time to get started living our happily ever after and embracing all that parenthood had to offer.

After getting all the paperwork squared away, packing up our belongings and thanking the hospital staff for going above and beyond with our "situation", we walked out the front door of the hospital with our baby boy.

It was surreal. I can't believe they were just letting us walk out of the hospital with a child that we had no idea how to care for. Sure, I'd read some parenting books, we took a class, but that was all theoretical. Now we had to keep this tiny human alive.

We walked to the car and put his tiny body into the car seat. It dwarfed him, and we had no idea whether we'd put him in correctly. Sure, we'd tested it out on a teddy bear after we had the seat fitted (no joke), but ted was much bigger (and squishier). In a moment of panic, I ran back into the hospital to see if someone would help us and check whether our little miracle was safely secured. They told us due to legalities; they weren't permitted to help us. So completely bizarre that they are okay with the possibility of sending a baby into a car unsecured, but are scared to check and risk being sued. So, we drove out of the hospital regardless and made the two-hour trek home from the hospital. It was the most nerve-wracking experience. I even sat in the back seat to make sure Luca was ok.

The next few weeks were like a dream. From everything people had told us, we were expecting the first few weeks to be hell. We'd told all our friends and family to give us a couple of weeks to settle in before visiting. We needed that time to bond with Luca and get to know him from scratch. I was still sensitive to the fact that we were strangers to him. So, we bunkered down.

It was during this time that a national morning show was holding a Christmas photo competition. I can't even remember if there was a prize, to be honest. However, we had just had a newborn baby photoshoot and received back the photos. They were divine. My favourite was a picture of Luca propped up with his head on his hands, a reindeer hat placed gently on his little head, his squishy cheeks in all their glory. Yes, I was a proud Mumma. So, we sent the picture into the morning show with a short blurb about how he came to be, and the fact that he was our little Christmas miracle.

The network jumped on it and emailed us immediately, wanting to do a segment on our story. We were shocked, terrified, but so excited and proud at the prospect. It moved so fast that I never really had time to process it. Renee was on board if we were ok with it. To be honest, I was still floating on cloud nine and was thrilled that someone else thought that we had a beautiful story.

It wasn't until the time was scheduled in our diary for camera crews to arrive at our house, that reality began to set in. Was I ready for this? For our story, still so raw, to be put out there for public scrutiny? I knew how horrible people could be through social media and how the media could twist a story to their advantage. I wasn't entirely comfortable putting ourselves out there to be judged. So, we cancelled the story.

Looking back, this was a good move. All it would have taken is for one or two people to be negative, and it would have pushed me down a spiral. My fear was that religious or other groups would stand up and say that if it didn't happen naturally, then it was god's or the universe's way of saying you don't deserve a baby.

If I'm completely honest, I didn't want to put it out there because I still wasn't comfortable with our story. I knew it was a lovely feel-good one; however, I still had a lot of unresolved issues. I hadn't made peace with the fact that we had to go down this path in the first place. Luca is now five years old, and I've only just worked through the resentment and disappointment in the process of writing this book.

Today I completely embrace where we came from, the path we went down, the emotions I felt, and the person I became in the process. What other people think of my story is of no consequence to how I feel about it. But back then, I didn't stand a chance.

There are a lot of things I would have done differently.

I can see now that my fertility journey consumed me. I had so much fear around what it meant about me and what other people would think. When you're in the thick of it, it's hard to see anything else. But if I could go back to that fearful woman who started this journey, I would tell her that this is merely a chapter in an amazing story of her life. And embracing that part, owning it, and seeing it as just a small part of our story is completely freeing. It doesn't have to hold you back.

People will judge no matter what. But as long as you know you're on the right path, it's of no consequence.

And the more I think about our journey, the more silver linings I can see.

One of the benefits of using a surrogate was the fact that I didn't have any post-baby hormones running through my body. I was in complete control of my thoughts and emotions. Of course, I didn't fully appreciate this until 17 months later.

On day three of being home from the hospital with Luca, we were getting a little stir crazy. We had watched back to back series of Arrow and countless movies. I had read my fill of vampire romance fiction (totally my thing back then) and everything was set up in the nursery.

Most importantly, however, Craig and I were having sex. At this point I will have to apologise to my husband and mother and father in law - I know they will be cringing by now, but yes, I'm going to go there. For five years, sex had been a constant reminder of how we were broken. It had merely been a form of reproduction – something to have at specific times. But not anymore. It was no longer a chore, and was back in our lives as something to do for fun!

It felt like a weight had been lifted. It wasn't dreaded, and there was no pressure. And the end goal was an orgasm, not to get pregnant. Even during the nine months prior, when we knew we were pregnant and going to have a baby, it was still in the back of my mind every time we had sex (which wasn't very often, to be honest with you).

This process has a way of stripping back every little joy in your life, especially around sex, and turning it into an obligation. Every month we weren't pregnant was a reminder that we were flawed, and that we weren't doing it right even though the majority of the population could. It was a constant spotlight on the fact that sex did not equal a baby for us. From the moment you start trying to conceive, sex has a purpose, and that is to get pregnant. And the longer it took to get pregnant, the more I hated having sex. I know Craig did too. It was like a slap in the face each time.

I never fully realised the toll it had taken on us until Luca came home with us. We had our little miracle, a newborn baby in his bassinet in the next room. There was no obligation attached to sex now. We weren't trying to have a baby. And it was freeing. Like a weight had been lifted from our shoulders. Every thought in the morning was not dripped in fear of if we would ever become parents, and every thought at night was not sadness that it hadn't happened yet. While the full gravity of our situation and what we had been through hadn't left entirely, our day to day felt lighter. There was more space to breathe. And more importantly, we had reconnected.

We must be the only parents with a newborn who were having sex like we were newlyweds. Come to think of it; we didn't even have sex this much on our honeymoon. It brought us much closer, and now our little family was complete, we could finally get on with living out our happily ever after.

And that is how I came to find myself locked in our bathroom, peeing on a stick......

Chapter 7

WHAT DID I DO TO DESERVE THIS?

T he other day, Luca had a meltdown. As a five-year-old, tantrums aren't uncommon; however, this one was different. It got my attention - the intensity of it scared me a little. I can't remember what even started it, but it ended in Luca standing in the middle of the room and just screaming like a banshee. His face went beet red; he was shaking, and tears were streaming down his cheeks. His body was rigid, his fists clenched, his mouth was wide open, with his head tilted to the sky. He was angry. Really angry, and this was the only way he was equipped to get it out.

After my initial shock, I watched him. He was clearly struggling to get out his anger, but what he was doing was working. After he finished, I quietly knelt and opened my arms.

He walked over, exhausted from his rant, and came in for a cuddle. I asked him if he was ok, and he quietly nodded. And then we went on our way.

Don't get me wrong; I'm not a poster child for parenting - our encounters sometimes end in me getting angry and yelling back. But he caught me on a calm day, so I was able to observe what was happening to his little body.

While in some situations, this may be considered bad behaviour, I could completely relate to his anger and inability to get it out.

I spent most of my fertility journey angry. That's seven years of pent up anger without knowing how to release it (because screaming and throwing a tantrum is socially unacceptable for a woman in her late 30's). Eventually, it catches up with you. And one day, it could be the slightest thing that pushes you over the edge.

Luca's outburst reminded me of a particular moment which I would have to describe as one of my top five ANGRY moments. The unjustness of it still evokes a physical reaction in me.

In this moment, I felt like ripping someone's head off. I was so mad – like pacing, throwing a tantrum, ugly crying mad.

What was so frustrating was the fact that my anger wasn't directed at a particular person. So there was no physical object that my feelings were targeted toward. I was angry at life in general.

Of course, no one would have known how angry I was by looking at me. Inside me was a hurricane on a path to self-destruction. It felt like I was about to combust spontaneously. Imagine a pot of boiling water with the lid on. But I kept that lid on tight and turned inward. I couldn't talk to anyone about it for fear that the lid would come off and everyone around me, including myself, would get scalded.

I was furious at God, the Universe or whatever higher power was at work here, and was convinced this had to be some sort of sick joke. Surely, I would wake up, and it would all be a dream. Or at any moment, Ashton Kutcher would walk into the room, and it would be an episode of Punked.

By then, Luca was six weeks old. We were still in that newborn euphoric stage. He was a dream baby and slept a lot, so we were starting to relax into parenthood. It was a bit surreal, and we still had to pinch ourselves that this was our new life. By this stage, Craig had gone back to work, and my new reality was setting in. I was braving it and going for walks along the water by myself with our beautiful boy.

We knew that Luca would be an only child. Don't get me wrong, deep down we had always wanted two children; however, Renee was clear that this was a one-time gig. And we were so lucky even to have one child, that it wasn't a big deal. There were so many couples out there who would kill to have what we did, so we were grateful for our one little miracle. Plus, there is no way we'd be able to go through that journey twice – emotionally or financially.

So that door was shut - firmly.

Have you heard the saying "When one door shuts, another one opens"?

I don't even remember how it happened (well, of course, I know HOW it happened), but I don't recall how I got to the point of peeing on a stick. I have no idea what even made me consider that being pregnant was a possibility given a board of doctors had diagnosed me as infertile. But here I was, sitting on the toilet in our bathroom, waiting for the verdict.

I had been in this position many times before. I should have bought shares in pregnancy test corporations given the number of tests I had purchased over the years we were trying to fall pregnant. But it was always such a heart-breaking experience – that moment of hope as you set your timer for two minutes and just pray for that second line to appear. Squinting, leaving it just a little bit longer in case it just needed more time. And then that feeling of deep disappointment in the pit of your stomach when you realise that the second line isn't going to appear, no matter how long you sit and stare at it. Walking away and checking it a couple of hours later, then throwing it in the trash, still wondering whether it was a faulty test. I was familiar with that feeling. It was soul-destroying.

What I wasn't familiar with was a second line appearing. So, you can imagine my surprise and bewilderment when it happened. I didn't tell Craig what I suspected or that

I was going to the shop to purchase a pregnancy test. There was no need to bring him along on this painful journey yet again. I sat there for the next few excruciating hours waiting for him to come home. I kept on wandering into the bathroom to make sure that the second line hadn't disappeared. I did another test, just to make sure. I practised over and over in my head what I would say when he eventually arrived home from work.

By the time he walked through the front door, I was busting out of my skin. I shoved the pregnancy test into his face and said, "I'm pregnant!". Probably not the most delicate way to announce a pregnancy. We both sat there in complete shock. I think the words "holy shit" were muttered quite a few times.

Here we were with a newborn baby that we had fought so hard to conceive, and now we had another one on the way.

FUCK??!!

We had just stepped off a five-year roller coaster ride and spent copious amounts of money only to fall pregnant naturally.......accidentally.

Renee still had the stitches in her stomach from her caesarean section for goodness sake. I felt so guilty – we put her through two years on the emotional IVF roller coaster, a miscarriage, and her body through nine months of pregnancy. As it turned out, I was quite capable of doing it myself.

How did this happen?

I have no fucking idea. I did nothing different consciously. I didn't start eating pineapple by the truckload, take a magic pill or cut something out of my diet. I didn't say a specific affirmation, buy a good luck charm, or do a particular meditation or yoga session.

But subconsciously, everything changed. I was no longer a prisoner to infertility. After being branded with that INFERTILE label for five years, I had finally escaped the stigma attached to it. I was living my life outside the chains that had kept me captive for all those years. A little dramatic? Perhaps. But that's exactly what happened. I wasn't consumed in anger and how unfair it was that other people fell pregnant on the pill, while I was trying for what seemed like a lifetime. I wasn't focused on what I didn't have; I was focused on what I DID have.

My stress levels had reduced significantly given the fact that I was on maternity leave. I had finally given my mind and body the space it had been desperate for. I wasn't punishing myself for what my body couldn't do - I cut myself some slack. I was no longer the woman who was childless; I was Jen.

I know this may piss you off. We're all searching for that magic pill because it's so much easier to swallow, than stop and think about the emotional toll this journey takes on us. We spend so much time trying to convince everyone around us that we're fine, and we're strong, and that this is merely a process, that in turn, we convince ourselves too. So, we end up pretending we're ok and avoid all talk of how we're feeling. In reality, we're scared of taking that lid off our emotions for fear of what we'll find inside. We figure the emotional toll this is taking on us will all be over when we have a baby, so we just want to tick the box and move to the next stage as quickly as possible.

But that is exactly what happened to me. The heavy emotional burden that I'd been carrying around on my shoulders that was previously so crippling lifted a little. Not entirely, but enough for me to breathe again.

So back to our current reality. It was surreal. It was a blur. We were in shock – I think I already said that. We were happy and terrified at the same time.

I remember going for my first blood test to confirm the result officially. I had a newborn baby in the pram beside me. The nurse just looked from me to Luca, utterly bewildered and stated – that's not physically possible. Yes – I know. We were the exception. I'd heard stories of a friend of a friend, or a cousin of an aunt who this had happened to. It's the sort of thing that happens to other people. But not us.

I used to get so caught up on statistics and probabilities and averages and think "this could never happen to me". But the truth is that I was the exception so many times that I know I'm not average anymore. Anything is possible. I don't have to be the rule, just because that's what makes everyone around me feel comfortable. Sometimes doctors get it wrong. Sometimes we get it wrong, despite our best attempts to always be right. And that can be a good thing.

When we told our family our news, they were so happy – they cried, we cried. This was real. No one could believe it – especially us.

So, we started planning for two children. Two children under one, that is. What would we do with our pram – we had only purchased a single? We'd have to get another camera for our baby monitor. Another car seat. Would I bother going back to work? Where would the new baby sleep?

We started dreaming again. I couldn't wait to feel my baby grow inside me and experience all the things I had missed out on with Luca. Maybe life wasn't so cruel. Perhaps the odds weren't stacked against us, and we weren't so flawed. I wrapped myself up in a blanket of hope. All was right with the world once again.

Nine weeks later, our fantasy and the false sense of security came crashing down around us. That all too familiar feeling of dashed hope and the unfairness of life was thrust in our faces. We were booted off our fertility roller coaster. Again.

FUCK!!!!!!!

As quickly as it happened, it was taken away. At our six week scan, they told us our baby was smaller than it should be, and the heartbeat was a little slow. We had blood tests, and it showed that my levels weren't increasing at the rate they were supposed to. Dread, devastation with a glimmer of hope underneath had returned.

I didn't want to be here. In limbo yet again. I was waiting to see whether the pregnancy would continue or whether I would have a miscarriage. I tried to focus my energy into being a loving mum for Luca, taking care of him and finally revelling in the happiness that he had brought into our lives. But it didn't work no matter how hard I tried.

A week later, we went for another scan, which confirmed there was no heartbeat. We were devastated. And I was so fucking angry. What had I done to deserve this? I didn't think I was a bad person, but the fertility gods had undoubtedly decided to screw me over in a big way.

Our doctor suggested if our baby didn't pass on its own over the next couple of days, we should present at the emergency room of our local hospital to be treated. I approached every trip to the bathroom with trepidation, and after zero movement, we headed to the hospital.

The emergency room was filled with unsavoury characters, and I could see sickness all around me. We walked up to the admissions desk and told them my situation. They gave me a number and told me to wait. After what seemed like an eternity, I had to explain my situation to yet another doctor. After what seemed like another eternity, they ushered me into an empty cubicle with thin curtains surrounding it. It did little to muffle the sound of patients all around me, in all states of sickness. I just kept on thinking; I'm not sick, I'm having a miscarriage.

I couldn't bear the thought of subjecting Luca to the germs and sickness all around us, so I encouraged Craig to take him home and told him that I would call if anything changed.

Sometime later, a student nurse came in and put a cannula in my arm. I had no idea why, given the fact that they hadn't told me what was happening, however, I was utterly drained and succumbed to whatever came next. The student nurse made several attempts to put the needle in my arm and finally found what he was looking for. I don't know whether it was the fragile state I was in, but it hurt a LOT. The pain in my arm matched the pain inside me. So, I laid in that bed, cold and alone, and silently cried. I couldn't believe I was back here again - rock bottom.

Every time a new doctor came in, I had to explain my situation. It never got any easier. Eventually, they told me that the Early Pregnancy Assessment Unit, which was where I was supposed to be was closed that day. I just wanted it to be over, but sadly it wasn't happening today. They told me they'd get someone to call me to make an appointment, took the cannula out of my arm, and sent me on my way.

The next couple of weeks were a blur.

We waited as time stood still. It's like that little foetus couldn't survive, but it didn't want to exit my body. Nothing happened, so a week later, they decided to induce a miscarriage, which is one of the most painful things I've ever experienced – both physically and mentally. I was so drugged up on painkillers that I couldn't tell whether my pain was in my body or my heart and soul. I remember laying in bed, in the dark, just waiting and desperate for it to be over.

Up until then, I thought I knew sadness and anger. It turns out I didn't – I hadn't even touched the surface of those emotions until I was mourning the loss of a baby, with a newborn in my arms. A newborn that we had fought so hard to get. What was supposed to be our happily ever after, was tainted by yet another loss.

I was emotionally spent and completely raw.

I was furious because we had just stepped off that five-year roller coaster, only to be dragged back on it, and then get pushed off again. What kind of sick world do we live in? I didn't want to get back on the roller coaster in the first place for Christ sakes. It was laughable (in a crazy hysterical joker kind of way).

I knew what I was going through at the time felt huge, and the gravity of the situation still sits with me today, as I put these words together with tears streaming down my face. So how does someone force themselves to get out of bed each day, get dressed and continue to put one foot in front of the other? How do you continue to function in a world that has completely let you down? You just do. You switch off and go into autopilot mode. And do what you have to do.

It changed me. You see, back then, I was a big believer that everything happens for a reason. So, I couldn't fathom what possible reason there was for me falling pregnant and then having a miscarriage. Surely life couldn't be so cruel.

Just recently, however, I read a book by Rachel Hollis and something she said resonated with me. She talks about her brother committing suicide and explains that at that moment, she threw out the saying that "everything happens for a reason". There can be no reason for a tragic event. But, she pointed out, there is a lesson in everything that happens. You just have to look for it.

Looking back now, I can see the lesson.

Up until then, I had only experienced a fraction of what Renee had gone through when she'd had her miscarriage. Now I knew the whole lot. If I didn't realise she was an Angel by now, this moment pushed it over the edge. She went through this for us. It was only an emotional loss for us, but add the physical loss into the mix, and you have a complete recipe for disaster. And yet she picked herself up, dusted herself off and tried again for us.

So, I used that as inspiration. I spent a week being angry and feeling sorry for myself, and then I pushed it down.

What I have learnt over the years, and especially from this experience is that we can endure pain long after we think we're at our limit.

So just like I had done so many times before, I picked myself up, dusted myself off, and got on with it. After all, I had a gorgeous baby to look after and appreciate. I had so much to be grateful for. There would be someone who would kill to be in our position of having a baby, and I owed it to them to push forward. So I did.

Chapter 8

SOPHIE: THE WHOLE NINE YARDS

So life went back to normal.

To be honest with you, we'd had so many changes in our lives over the past year; when I say it went back to normal, I have no idea what normal was.

Our next focus was on adopting Luca. I know, it sounds ridiculous. This little boy was our flesh and blood, had been living with us for the last five months, and was still not legally our son. We had a birth certificate that said Renee and Nathan were his mum and dad.

It wasn't from lack of trying though. Under the Surrogacy Act in our state at the time, we had to wait at least 28 days from birth to lodge the paperwork. And I was keen to get the paperwork filed as quickly as possible.

The day before Luca was born, I rang our solicitor to get the ball rolling. The process of adoption was just as drawn out and even more expensive than setting up the original surrogacy agreements. It once again included lawyers on both sides, counselling for all parties concerned, copious amounts of paperwork and affidavits, and ended up with us in court. We faced delays over Christmas with the courts being closed, and then our solicitor's office being closed, and even the counsellor. There were a million phone calls back and forth. I pushed, I followed up, I was desperate to get this over with as soon as possible.

I'll never forget our day in court. I tossed and turned the night before, afraid that we'd sleep through the alarm. We arrived early and met Renee and Nathan at the coffee shop underneath the courthouse. I could hardly eat; I was so nervous. And there was that familiar feeling of self-doubt in the pit of my stomach. That little voice of disappointment that told me once again, I was just a bystander in this process. I once again had to prove that I was worthy of being a mum. My smile that day was completely fake. I was even a little angry. But mostly I was scared because this was out of my control. In my head, I knew that this was just another step in a very regulated process that was all about minimising risk. But in my heart, it was another person saying that this little boy wasn't truly ours. It was another time we had to stand up (this time in a court of law), prove that we were worthy of being parents, relinquish control to another person, and fight to make this happen. To be honest, I was sick of fighting and pushing. The judge would ultimately determine whether we were allowed to be the legal guardians of our child. We were at the mercy of our solicitor and the legal system.

As if things weren't stressful enough, Renee's lawyer was running late to court, which gave us absolutely no confidence in her ability to make this a smooth process. It was like an episode of Suits, except Harvey Spector wasn't fighting for us. Maybe if he was, it would make this worthwhile, and I could forgive him for being late.

We all walked into the sterile and overwhelming courtroom and took our places at two separate tables. It was like we were opposing each other instead of fighting for the same thing. It was quite ironic; a lawyer represented us, another lawyer represented Renee, and we were footing the bill for both. Our whispers echoed in the empty room, and my hands were shaking once again. There were none of the usual jokes thrown around. We knew this was serious. This was the last step in the process, and none of us wanted to have to come back here.

It was a completely surreal moment; our solicitor stating our case, and Renee's lawyer (when she eventually arrived) stating theirs. We held our breath as the judge considered the evidence and finally made the judgement that yes, we could be granted legal custody and guardianship of Luca.

Five months after he came into our lives, we officially adopted our child. I was officially a mother in the eyes of the law.

It was a huge relief, so we celebrated. Amongst the hustle and bustle of the city where everyone was scurrying off to work, we sat drinking champagne at 10 am celebrating yet another milestone. Responsible parenting? Who cares! We'd all earned that glass of champagne, and the court couldn't take it back. After the hype, we all went back home as if nothing had happened, and life returned to "normal".

For the next few months, we were absorbed by our little family. I was loving my time off work and walking down to the bay with Luca in the pram, soaking up the sunshine and living our happily ever after.

There were still moments that reminded me we had a different story, however. I had joined a mother's group shortly after Luca was born to connect with other first-time mums. The conversations usually revolved around breast-feeding or childbirth, of which I had zero experience. I smiled, nodded and listened to their stories, but couldn't contribute. It hurt that I still felt like an outsider. I had a beautiful story to tell, which was met by curiosity and amazement. Nevertheless, in the back of my mind, I wondered when the normal experience would begin. When my story wouldn't feel like a part was missing.

We went for weekends away, attended weddings where we rocked Luca to sleep in the pram and tucked him safely behind our table while we celebrated with our friends. Sundays were spent taking him to swimming lessons and catching up with friends for breakfast afterwards. He didn't cramp our style much at all.

Don't get me wrong, parenthood is and will always be the hardest thing I have done in my life. I had read all the baby books and had a feeding and sleep schedule to keep track, but there was no pattern. He had trouble feeding, so we switched baby bottles and formula a million times. It was harder than I thought it was going to be; however, given the shit fight we had been through to get here, it was a walk in the park.

For me, the biggest struggle was realising that I couldn't control things anymore. As if my path so far wasn't message enough, it has taken me all this time (ok, I'm a slow learner) to realise the more you push it, the more resistance you'll get. But driving to get what I wanted was all I knew. I was taught from a young age that if you want something, you go out and get it. And the harder you work at it, the more likely you are to succeed.

Which is the EXACT opposite for infertility. I couldn't control the outcome no matter how hard I tried - and I tried!! That's exactly what sent me into a tailspin. But all those years I was focusing on the thing I couldn't control as opposed to the things I could. I could control my diet, how much I exercised........and my mindset. But I couldn't see that. All I wanted to control was the result, and in life, we never get to control that. No wonder I got so frustrated!

The first six months of Luca's life had flown by. As my time on maternity leave came to an end, I had mixed emotions. Luca and I had formed a great little bond, and I was enjoying the lazy lifestyle that came with no pressure. After a career that was filled with deadlines, climbing the corporate ladder, managing a team and making stressful decisions, this was a refreshing change. My only goal each day was to keep him alive. But I needed something more.

So, I went back to work, and Craig went on paternity leave. It was tough leaving Luca given the fact that we'd gone through so much to get to this point. However, I'm a "do-er" and to be honest; I was looking forward to going back to a job where I had at least a little control. I was the chief financial officer, so if I asked my team or anyone else to do something, they did it. I craved the sense of achievement that came with reaching a goal, making a difference, and real purpose. For the previous six months, my life had been about baby formula, poop, sleep routines, and I was ready for a little more.

Don't get me wrong; I have the utmost respect for any woman who stays at home to raise their family. It seriously is the hardest job in the world. But I wanted more. It's taken me a long time to be able to say that without wavering or feeling guilty. I'm not sure whether it's because our path to get here was so long and heartbreaking, but I've always blamed money on me working. In truth, however, it's because I worked damn hard to get where I am. I thrive on achievement, targets, strategy and continual growth. At home, I was living the same day over and over again, and while Luca was thriving and growing, I wasn't.

I was welcomed back to work with open arms, flowers, chocolates and pictures of Luca all over my office. It was nice. And so, I settled into my life of being a working mum, receiving updates on Luca and Craig's adventures via text message and photos. I loved that they were forming a little bond, although at times I felt a little left out.

I've been sitting here wracking my brain and going through photos trying to pinpoint the moment our world started to tilt again, but I can't. I wish it were a monumental moment leading up to it, but it wasn't. Since my miscarriage, I knew in the back of my mind that a natural pregnancy was an option. Miraculously my body had figured out what it had been doing wrong for the last six years and had righted itself. But I wasn't purposefully trying. Don't get me wrong, estimating my ovulation date was an ingrained habit, and having sex around that date was always a goal, but it wasn't driving me. I never told Craig either. I didn't want to go back to the beginning where we had put so much pressure on ourselves. It wasn't pleasant, and to be honest, I would still have been happy with only one child. I kept thinking that there are others out there who would love to be in my situation, and I was so grateful.

Ok, I'm calling bullshit on myself. Who am I kidding?! Yes, I was secretly trying. Craig was oblivious given the fact that he was a stay at home dad at the time, so it was the furthest thing from his mind. So not only was I not telling Craig, but I wasn't admitting it to myself either. Because then there would be disappointment and pressure, and next thing you know I'd be back on that freaking fertility roller coaster.

The truth is I was so connected to my body from years of tracking, that it was an automatic response. Before we started trying to conceive, I had no idea what my cycle was or how my body worked. But over the years you watch out for signals, twitches in your ovaries, changes in patterns and new symptoms occurring. I understood my body better than anyone else, and every month there was a fraction of hope before my period arrived. But I was in denial because I did NOT want to get back on that ride. The thought made me feel a little sick actually.

While for most people a miscarriage is a sinking ship, for me it was a beacon of hope. I'd had a taste, and I was back on board. This time, however, I wasn't obsessed. The desperation wasn't there. If it didn't happen, I'd be ok. There was no timeframe or pressure, and no angst around sex.

While I was back at work, it wasn't the most important thing in my life. I wasn't trying to prove my worth. I left work on time and didn't bring the stress home with me.

Life just felt easy, calm and comfortable.

And it worked. My period was a week late, so you guessed it...... I found myself once again locked in my bathroom, peeing on a stick. And once again - those two magic little lines appeared.

YES!!!!

This time around, there was a mixture of excitement and fear. We were afraid to get our hopes up in case fate stepped in and robbed us of this experience yet again. But I figured we had a secret weapon this time. When

I had fallen pregnant eight months beforehand, I had started seeing Anne, our mother nature acupuncturist. By the time I saw her back then; however, it was too late.

But I had been going to see her every fortnight since then. Not only was it an opportunity for a little ME time, but with Luca, work and life in general, I needed a little balance and calming. And that is what Anne was for me. She was my safe haven; a place I could go and let my guard down. It was a form of release. At times I found myself crying on the 30-minute drive to go and see her - I thought I was going crazy until she explained it was my body anticipating the release.

I remember one particular session with her. It was a few months after my miscarriage. After an emotional week, I found myself once again crying in her treatment room. I think she could sense there was something that I was holding onto. She asked me if there was one thing I could have in this world, what would it be? My answer surprised me and made me feel guilty as hell. I wanted to have a baby myself. I wanted to carry it, grow it, feel it and nurture it. I felt as though I had been robbed of a really important experience. I had no idea I was holding this inside me. On reflection, I kept everything inside me so tight it's no wonder I was crying in most sessions. I felt guilty because I had no right to be so ungrateful. Renee had gone through so much to gift us with Luca, and I had a beautiful baby boy, and I still wasn't happy?

Looking back now, it seems so ridiculous - I felt guilty because I wanted to have a baby myself? Why should I feel guilty for wanting something that comes so easily and sometimes accidentally to others? But I did. I felt ashamed because there were people who would give anything to be in our position. And here's the thing – there will always be someone less fortunate in every stage of my life. But just because of that, it didn't mean my struggle wasn't valid.

I wish I could have seen it from that angle at the time. It is entirely possible to be grateful and want more at the same time. And while I was completely grateful for Luca, I still craved the full experience.

This time we didn't tell a soul that we were pregnant (well apart from Anne). Oh, and my best friend at the time. She had flown over from New Zealand as a surprise for my 39th birthday. A weekend of birthday celebrations with no wine involved was a hard sell. We'd hired a hotel room in the city for the night and organised to go out with some girlfriends for a "drink". I had to fake a hangover to explain why I wasn't drinking - such a stark contrast to our first pregnancy with Luca. I could no longer drink, and I had to hide the physical symptoms. I have no idea whether my girlfriends believed my excuse or not. I was secretly hoping that because they knew of my fertility issues, they wouldn't suspect a thing.

I remember waking up in the morning after my birthday celebrations feeling sick. To be honest, this wasn't unusual; however, it was usually a hangover. My sickness was a horrible, yet welcome feeling. I sat in the lobby eating salt and vinegar chips trying to settle my stomach. And that's how it was for the first trimester. I had morning sickness (and it doesn't just happen in the morning), I was constantly tired, and my breasts were sore. I spent the next few weeks sneaking crackers under my desk at work too.

I wrestled with my feelings - I swung from thinking how much this sucked to feeling completely grateful. I loved the sickness that a "real" pregnancy experience provided. I loved being tired, and I loved being sore. I kept on having to pinch myself.

Even today, when I hear other women complaining about their symptoms and how horrible their pregnancy was, I want to shake their shoulders. I want to tell them that there are worse things than feeling sick, tired and sore. I want to tell them that the feeling of NOT being pregnant every single month is more painful than any symptom they will ever experience on their nine-month journey. I want to tell them that carrying a child inside you is a complete blessing. AND I want to say to them that if they can't handle pregnancy, just wait for motherhood!!

If nothing else, my fertility journey prepared me for motherhood in the most extreme way. Infertility taught me patience, that I cannot control everything, to let go of that perfect picture in my head, stop planning so much, and that I need to ask for help. If you ask me, that is a course in parenting for beginners.

The day of our 12-week scan was terrifying. My morning sickness had subsided, and in the back of our minds, we were trying to prepare ourselves for the worst. Would there be a heartbeat? You could almost cut the tension with a knife.

I can tell you; the relief felt the moment that little blob and a jagged line appeared on the screen was intense. Gadoonk gadoonk gadoonk gadoonk. That magic sound echoed in our ears.

Every time I hear that sound, it gives me chills and makes tears well up in my eyes. The number of scans I went through with IVF, and every single time my insides were projected on that screen, I always scanned it for a baby and listened for a heartbeat. Even when it was during a stims cycle, and there was no possibility of pregnancy. It was a habit formed in those seven years and one I still have. Just the other day I went for an ultrasound check-up for some legions they had found on my ovaries 12 months earlier. As I was looking at the screen, I was holding my breath and searching for a heartbeat, despite knowing full well that I wasn't pregnant.

After the scan, we walked out of the room, relieved and elated and rang everyone we knew.

Our news was met with surprise and pure joy. We had our little miracle for a second time. Of course, there was a little confusion from those who were familiar with our story; however, we were used to complicated and having to explain ourselves.

When I broke the news to my team at work, I cried....... again. They were shocked, of course, but no one with a heart could begrudge me this opportunity. Typically when you announce your pregnancy, the question isn't HOW? That's pretty obvious. But in our case, it was a fair question. They wanted to know how this could happen, given our previous struggles. My response was usually….. it turns out I can after all!

I loved the second trimester. I loved what it was doing to my body - I felt energised. I was going to the gym still, walking along the bay and I watched my baby bump grow in wonder. I still miss that feeling today. I loved laying down and seeing and feeling my belly ripple with each kick. This is something I had only ever seen on a video with Luca, but now I was experiencing it myself. And that park scene in Notting Hill? Well, I was no Julia Roberts, and Craig was no Hugh Grant, but we had those moments.

At our 16 week scan, we found out we were having a little girl. I know we were both hoping for a girl given the fact that we had always thought that Luca would be wrapped in pink. Life has a funny way of working itself out.

We signed up for prenatal classes this time given this was my first real birth, and I hoped to breast-feed too. I relished every moment of the normal pregnancy experience and all the things I missed out on previously.

Halfway through the pregnancy, I was diagnosed with gestational diabetes. It threw me a curveball. And I must admit I was disappointed that I wouldn't be able to eat my way through a tub of Baskin Robbins peanut butter and chocolate ice cream. Still, in the end, it all worked out. I had been putting on a few extra unwanted kilos, so this forced me to eat healthily and monitor my blood sugar level. In hindsight it was a great thing - I finished the pregnancy with very little fat on my body. I was probably in better shape during the pregnancy (apart from the massive basketball in front) than I was beforehand.

In the last four weeks of my pregnancy, I found out that our little girl hadn't turned around. She was breech, and we were faced with the decision of turning her around, a painful and risky process, or leaving her in place and me having to have a planned caesarean. I wasn't a fan of the caesarean. I had wanted to be pregnant for so long, and I wanted the FULL experience. The labour, the lot! I know that sounds weird, but when you spend five years of your life craving being pregnant, being pregnant was the cake, and labour was like the icing on top. But there was no way we were going to put our little girl at risk either, just because the birth I had pictured in my head wasn't going to happen.

On reflection, it seems absurd that I had gotten to this point, and I still had a picture in my head of how I wanted things to go down. Surely by now, I would have learnt that with me and fertility - things would NEVER go the way I pictured. The only sure thing was that they wouldn't.

So, we booked ourselves in for a caesarean and planned our life around it accordingly.

My farewell at work and exit into maternity leave this time around was a little different. There was no hiding the fact that I was going off to have a baby. I was trying to wrap everything up because I knew that this time, with two children, I probably wouldn't have the time to help out while I was off work. I waddled out of the zoo on my last day, feeling completely exhausted and sick. By this stage, my diet consisted of icy poles and watermelon - I just couldn't fit anything else in.

The scans had revealed that I was going to give birth to a giant, and I must admit I was a little terrified given the fact that I'm usually a petite size eight. But at least I wouldn't have to push her out!

Looking back, I loved those last moments. Not at the time, but they are memories that I don't have with Luca. For him, our memories started on day one when he was placed into my arms. But with Sophie, I will always have a full story, and for that, I will be forever grateful.

I'd planned to have two weeks off before we became a family of four. But, once again, things didn't go the way I had planned. I finished work and went into labour four days later.

Of course, at the time, I had no idea I was in labour. Nothing can prepare you for what it feels like; I just knew I was uncomfortable. And more uncomfortable than normal given the fact that I had a baby inside me whose head was wedged under my rib cage. By 8 pm that night, I was starting to feel a fair bit of pain. By the time we went to bed, I was lying there unable to sleep. Of course, Craig was snoring softly beside me. When I poked him and told him I wasn't feeling well, he suggested I have a bath and promptly rolled back over into the land of nod.

So here I was, lying in a warm bath at 10 pm, still unable to find any comfort. I'd say at this point, all thoughts of being grateful for this opportunity went out the window. I am human, and I have my limits, and at the time, all I could think of was the pain. On reflection, this was the moment that it hit me. The magnitude of what Renee had gone through for us. If I hadn't gone through this whole process myself, I never would have appreciated the level of pain and sacrifice she had gone through for us. But now I do.

After waddling back to bed after my bath, I lay there staring at the wall, in a considerable amount of pain, with my husband still sleeping peacefully beside me. He's lucky at this point that I didn't smother him with a pillow. So, I nudged him and told him that I was in a lot of pain. He suggested I ring the hospital and find out what they thought, and once again rolled back over and started quietly snoring again.

The hospital suggested I come in. I must say, at this point, I gladly shook Craig awake and told him we were going to the hospital. We bundled our 17-month-old sleepy little Luca into the car and drove the 20 minutes up the road. On arriving, I limped out of the car and walked up to the entrance. By this stage, it was around 1 am, so there wasn't anyone to assist, just a phone on a wall.

Once inside, I shuffled my way to the maternity ward, in a haze of pain. They put me in a room and started taking my vitals and asking me questions. My usual reaction to intense pain is vomiting, so at this point, it was all coming out: watermelon and icy poles. After the routine examinations, the nurse came and put my hand on the lower part of my bulging belly. She quietly said, darling, you feel that movement there? Yes, I grimaced with my spew bag still tightly gripped in the other hand. That's a contraction - you're three centimetres dilated.

I turned to my husband who was at the end of the bed holding Luca - I TOLD YOU I WAS IN PAIN! I seethed at him. I think he was shocked. Later (after it was safe to speak) he revealed he thought I was being a little dramatic about the pain I was in at the time.

From there, it was a flurry of excitement. There was no way I could deliver naturally, so after about 10 minutes, they walked in and told me that the operating theatre was free, so we were going down to have a baby right now. WHAT??!!! I wasn't prepared for this. At this point, however, I just wanted the pain to be over.

It wasn't until they started wheeling me down the corridor that it hit me. I was going to have to do this alone. We didn't have time to call someone to look after Luca - our nearest relatives were an hour away. It was a complete blur and happened so fast I didn't have time to process it. Luckily, I'd been through the caesarean process with Renee, so I knew what to expect. The shoe was on the other foot this time though.

I remember when I was all prepped, epidural administered, lying on the cold, hard operating table, the nurse whispering in my ear - will anyone be joining us? In my head, I was explaining that, yes, I do have a husband, but he's upstairs with our other baby. Instead, I just shook my head – no - just me.

I have no idea how long it took, but they eventually placed a small baby wrapped in a blanket beside my head. Here's your baby, they said. I looked at her, nodded my head, and started shaking. I was freezing. If I'm completely honest, I didn't feel much of a connection to my baby either. I think I was in shock at how quickly everything had transpired. They whisked her away, and I was wheeled into recovery, where I remained shivering and alone.

*   *   *

Two babies. Two completely different experiences.

For Luca, I was completely conscious and alert. His entrance into the world was filmed, photographed, and had three family members present and celebrating his arrival. There were tears of joy. But it cost us five years, bucket loads of money and a million tears and heartbreak. And I had to sacrifice the full pregnancy experience I had dreamed of.

Sophie's was a blur. No photographs, fanfare and I was alone. I didn't cuddle her, get excited or cry tears of joy. I just nodded. But I got to experience her growing and moving inside me every step of the way and formed a bond from the very beginning.

As I'm sitting here writing this, I'm trying to think of what this all means. And therein lies the problem.

I have spent so much time over the years, focusing on why this was happening to me - searching for an answer to those questions. Why is it taking so long for me to fall pregnant when others find it so easy? Is it because I don't deserve to be a mum? Did I do something wrong?

Overthinking and analysing everything and getting wrapped up in what everyone else was doing around me or what they thought.

What I DO know is that right now, downstairs are two beautiful children. They are sitting on the couch watching Ratatouille, oblivious to the fact that I'm over here, debating which of their path to pregnancy and births was better.

And at the end of the day, it doesn't matter. They don't care. And if they don't care, why should I?

Chapter 9

THE SLOW EXHALE:
EMBRACING OUR TRUTH

New Year's Eve started like any other day.

Apart from being on holidays, we woke up at 6 am (children have absolutely no concept of sleep-ins!) had breakfast, and went downstairs for a walk along the beach. We were staying in an apartment with my sister, brother in law and their three children, so we spent some time with them. I sat on the balcony overlooking the ocean, but I was feeling a little off centre. I was going down a path with a business I was developing that I didn't feel completely aligned with, and I was also bloody tired. It had been a hectic year.

Little did I know that this day would be the catalyst for major changes in my life.

Mid-morning, we packed up our belongings, jumped in the car and made the hour drive down south. We were spending New Years with Craig's family – his mum, dad, sister Renee, brother in law Nathan and their two children. We were looking forward to it.

For the last couple of months, Luca and Sophie had been obsessed with babies. Quite a few of their friends were becoming big sisters and brothers, and a couple of their teachers at child care were pregnant. On more than one occasion, they had told me there was a baby in my tummy. I usually laughed it off, but I do believe that children have a sixth sense about these things. In the lead up to one particular day, I had been feeling quite uncomfortable and bloated. They wore me down with their claims that there was a baby in my tummy, and in the back of my head, I went back to my mid-20's when the psychic predicted I would have three children from two pregnancies.

I also know it was utterly absurd given the fact that shortly after Sophie was born, Craig had a vasectomy. Yep, that's another experience where we sat in the waiting area looking at each other thinking – did you EVER think we'd be sitting here getting this done. For seven years, we had struggled to fall pregnant, and now we were taking additional precautions to make sure that the door was firmly closed. Completely bizarre how life works!

Anyhow, Craig had never gone back to test that the procedure had been effective. Plus, I had heard stories of people still falling pregnant afterwards. From my experience, we were an excellent chance to be an exception to this rule as well.

So, there I was, it was almost 10 years from when we had first started trying to conceive, peeing on a bloody stick again. I was feeling hopeful, excitement and terror all at the same time. My little cherubs were growing up way too quickly, so another baby meant that I could hold onto this phase of my life a little longer.

Don't worry - there isn't another twist to this story - we're near the end. The test came back negative; however, to this day, I still approach every month with trepidation, hope and excitement. It was such an ingrained habit for so many years that I always get a pang of disappointment every month when my period arrives.

Anyway, back to the car trip and the kid's obsession with babies in tummies. They were chatting in the back seat to each other about who had a baby in their belly, and what it was like when they were babies.

Craig and I had every intention of telling Luca the truth about his conception. During the counselling sessions at the beginning of our surrogacy process, it was strongly encouraged, and at the time we didn't think it would be a big deal. But right now? Already? He was only four years old at the time, and we were both worried that he wouldn't understand.

I, on the other hand, was worried that it would mean something. That it would change things, that he would look at me differently, that he would feel left out - different. My sister Kim was adopted, and it was an issue for her, so I used that as a guidepost. I was scared of speaking it out loud, of putting it all out on the table. I was scared that he would love me a little less.

This was the first time since we had gotten off that roller coaster that I realised perhaps I hadn't made peace with our journey. That I was still embarrassed, and it still hurt.

So while we weren't ready to tell Luca the truth, I wasn't going to lie to him about it. He must have sensed we were dodging his question about when he was in my tummy. He would mention it, and we would shrug it off. But he had us trapped. We were in the car and couldn't avoid him or escape to a different room. And he was like a dog with a bone. Until......"Mummy, do you remember when I was in your tummy?"

It was like slow motion. I glanced at Craig, who had a look of "oh crap" on his face, raised my eyebrow, took a deep breath and simply stated, "Well you weren't in my tummy because it was broken, so Aunty Renee had you in her tummy." It was like time stood still. I could tell Craig was holding his breath too. We were waiting for the verdict. Would there be more questions? Would he be upset?

I looked back at him in his car seat, and he simply shrugged, said ok, and asked, "Was Sophie in your tummy?". Oh, crap – another deep breath in and "Yes, mummies tummy was fixed by then, so Sophie was in my tummy". Once again, he looked at me, shrugged and said "Ok", and kept on nattering away about inconsequential topics. All the while, Craig and I were breathing a sigh of relief.

When we reached Craig's mum and dads place, we unloaded the kids and the bags and settled in. Renee, Nathan and the boys were already there, so we grabbed a well-earned, much-needed glass of wine and sat down.

I'll never forget this moment. It was the moment I truly felt I could embrace our story and let go of the embarrassment and shame surrounding the lengths we had to go to, to become parents.

In the car, before we'd come inside, I'd told Luca that he should probably thank Aunty Renee for having him in her tummy. He thought that was a great idea too. So, when we were sitting at the table with Renee and Robyn (Craig's mum), Luca walked around to Renee and in his softly spoken voice said – "Thank you for having me in your tummy."

Renee's eyes went wide, and she looked at me "Did he just say what I think he said?". "Yes", I said. I was bursting with pride at my little boy and the way he took the news that he had been in someone else's tummy, while Sophie had been in mine. I had tears in my eyes as a wave of relief washed over me. Well, that started the waterworks. Renee was in tears; Robyn was in tears. Luca looked a little confused as he was hugged by all of us a little tighter than ever before.

At that point, Craig walked over and asked what was happening and why we were all crying. You missed it – one of the greatest moments of my life.

I exhaled for the first time in what felt like a long time. I paused and took the time to look around me and absorb all we had achieved – two beautiful children. A family bonded forever with an amazing story. Now, I know that all mothers should think their children are gorgeous, but mine are the cutest you'll ever meet. Luca is a sweet-natured, gentle, caring and sensitive little boy. Sophie is timid, headstrong, a complete entertainer, polite one minute and ruthless the next. And we did it. We created these two beautiful souls who are the perfect combination of both Craig and me.

It wasn't easy; it was the toughest thing I have EVER endured. It completely changed me in ways I'm only starting to discover now.

I have spent almost 10 years hung up on the path that was forced upon me to get where I am. I have resented those around me that had it so easy. I have spent so much time wondering whether this wasn't meant to be – the fact that I couldn't fall pregnant and that we faced roadblocks at every avenue that we encountered. That maybe this wasn't "God's plan".

But most of all, I've cared about what other people thought. Everyone we tell our story to is in awe of our journey. However deep down I have always wondered what they're thinking. In reality, I've been projecting my feelings onto them.

We care so much about what the people around us think, instead of the people that matter. And within a couple of hours on New Year's Eve, it was all shattered. It didn't matter what Sally down the road thought. It didn't matter whether a religious group frowned upon our method. What mattered was what that little boy thought. How did he feel? Did he accept it? Did he still feel just as loved as any other child who had a "normal" story?

And he was ok. To this day he still hasn't forgotten. He always talks about when Aunty Renee had him in her tummy. And when we all catch up now, instead of feeling that fear and doubt creep in when I see them interact. I feel love, joy and gratitude. I love it when he hugs her, and I see the way she looks at him, with complete adoration. The moments they share aren't just those between an aunty and a nephew; they are so much more. They represent the challenges we overcame, the lowest points in our life where we didn't think we could endure any more, but we got back up anyway. The fight for what we knew we were entitled to, and never giving up.

This journey changed all of our lives.

Owning this chapter in my story has set me free. It's like a weight has finally lifted from my shoulders. One that had been suffocating me and hanging over my head for a decade.

And if I could turn back the hands of time and choose a normal path. One that didn't have the ups and downs, the exorbitant amount of money spent, the tears and heartache. I wouldn't. I'd choose our path 100 times over.

Because it's not about the journey, it's about who you become in the process.

Chapter 10

HEALING: ACCEPTANCE, FORGIVENESS AND LOVE.

True healing can only begin with acceptance, forgiveness, and most of all, true love. Writing my story has been the catalyst for my healing. During this process, I have fallen apart and pieced myself back together again. I am so proud of my determination and resilience throughout our journey. And while the injustice of being thrown into the realms of infertility still creates ripples of passionate indignation inside me, I don't feel like I was a victim to it. I have never been so grateful for everything in my life as I am at this very moment. And even though there are things I wish I could change; I have forgiven myself for being unable to see the rabbit hole before I slipped down it. For being so driven and focused that I couldn't see the damage I was causing to myself and those around me.

Very few people can say that they love themselves out loud without choking on the words. Without feeling selfish or egotistical. And it makes me a little sad that it has taken me over 40 years to get to the point where I genuinely admire not only the person I am today, but the person I have been all along.

This part of the story is for me. It may be considered a little self-indulgent; however, I think I deserve it. While I can't turn back the hands of time and rewrite history, nor embrace her and let her cry in my arms, I can write a letter to that naive 33-year-old who was about to embark on the journey of her life. I can tell her that it's going to be ok, to help her shoulder the heavy burden of infertility. This letter is the doorway to healing, and once I walk through it, I will finally be free to embark on my next journey. So, stay tuned.

Dear Jen,

You are the most incredible and bravest person I have ever known. Not to mention funny, honest and completely real. An exterior of strength, yet caring, gentle and kind on the inside. You are beautiful from the inside out and deserve every happiness that comes your way. I know that you'll brush this off and it will even make you feel a little uncomfortable reading these words. But I need you to know that. What you have endured up until now is enough to bring even the strongest of people to their knees. But you got back up after every setback and have become more resilient and determined as a result. You are a force to be reckoned with, and I am so proud of the woman you have become.

I'm telling you this now, not to blow smoke up your ass, but because you are about to embark on a journey that is tougher than any you have encountered before. I know, right?!! It will require strength and resilience beyond your comprehension. You will get knocked down so many times. You will travel to the darkest of places and cry a river of tears. Your heart will break so badly that at times, you will wonder whether you will ever be able to put it back together again.

But don't be afraid, because you are strong and you are a fighter. We are never given more than we can handle, and there will be times when you doubt whether you can lift the load and stand back up. You can. Your strength and determination, while some may consider annoying and stubborn, is what will save you time and time again.

There will be moments when you feel like the whole world is against you. You will question whether you did something wrong and whether you deserve the life that you have always dreamed of. You have done nothing wrong. You do deserve it. And you will get there.

You will question who you are, time and time again. There will be days when you don't even recognise the person staring back at you in the mirror. She is still there. But you need to start taking care of yourself, or you will lose yourself to this journey. And I don't mean taking extra bubble baths or getting a massage, although you should definitely do that too. I mean being gentle with yourself. You will need all of your strength to get through this, so take a break when you need to. Recharge. Stop pushing and trying to prove that you're worthy because you already are. Stop running so hard and punishing yourself if you don't live up to your ridiculously high expectations of yourself. Stop being so mean to yourself. I mean it - stop that shit!

And while we're at it, stop trying to control everything. It's fucking exhausting just thinking about how much you push yourself, how fast you run, and how many balls you have in the air to ensure it all works out perfectly. Life is precious; we all know that. But every moment doesn't have to be productive. Sit on your ass girl! Put your feet up and enjoy the fruits of your labour. Take *one day and one step at a time. Let me tell you now; you cannot control this outcome no matter how hard you try. Release your grip a little. Take a step back. Breathe. Have faith in yourself and trust that things will work out exactly how they're supposed to in the end.*

I know that hard work has gotten you to where you are right now. And I am so proud of all that you have achieved to date. You have everything that you have ever wanted, and it wasn't just luck that got you here. Your work ethic and the way your mind works is admirable. But that attitude and approach won't work this time. The harder you push, the further it will move away from you, and the more you will lose yourself.

You will begin to think that your sole purpose in life is to have a baby and that your life has no meaning without one. That you are worthless if you never become a mum. And the longer it takes, the more determined you will become. The less whole you will feel. You will sacrifice anything and everything to get what you want. But if you're not careful, it will come at a considerable cost........being YOU. And I can tell you now that your purpose in life is so much bigger than just becoming a mum.

You will wonder whether your struggles are a sign that it's just not meant to be. Just because your journey is hard, it doesn't mean that you won't be a good mum. I can tell you that you are going to be an incredible mum. This journey will teach you patience, gratitude, and love like you never knew was possible. And this is exactly what makes a good mum to her very core. This journey will teach you to be the best mum you can be. Of course, you won't see this for quite some time. I'm only just realising it now as I'm writing this letter to you.

The longer you're on this journey, the more you will want to shut off from the rest of the world and pull the covers over your head. I don't blame you. What you're about to go through is monumental, and the emotional toll will be too much to comprehend at times. So you will put up your walls and try to work through it by yourself. And given your history in dealing with emotions, you will try to put a lid on this to save yourself (and those around you). You will want to bury your head in the sand and push the pain down inside you. You will distract yourself by focusing on the next step, and you will tell yourself that this will all disappear when you get to the end, and you get your baby.

I wish I could tell you otherwise, but it won't work this time. You can't run away from something this big AND the grief and pain you're feeling won't just magically disappear when you have your baby. I'm sorry, but you will need to face every single set back instead of holding it in. Running and pushing won't work either.

Cry. It is ok to cry. It is also ok to say how shit this is. It doesn't make you weak, or negative, or a whinger. I don't know how much shit you need to go through to prove to yourself that you're strong. That you are no longer that broken and weak 20-year-old woman who was treated poorly by a man. You have nothing to be scared of anymore. You are going to be ok.

This journey is not going to go according to the way you had pictured it when you were younger. I'm sorry. Your story won't be one filled with rainbows and unicorns. It won't be a fairy-tale that you get to tell your children when you tuck them into bed at night. It will be SO much more than that. Yours will be a story of inspiration and resilience and hope. It will give people a whole different perspective and move them to tears. Yours will be a story that they will never forget. And when you tell your children, they will know that you fought for them every step of the way. That you never stopped trying to find them. And that they are special and loved and treasured more than anything in this world.

There is no need to be ashamed, nor is there anything wrong with you. Owning and accepting your story will set you free.

I love you. Now you need to start loving you too.

Xx

Appendix

THE LESSONS

Holy cow, what a ride that was! Does anyone else need a glass of wine after that? Just me?

I feel like I have lived a thousand lives all squeezed into a decade. I can't believe that this is my story. Sure, I wrote the words, but that's the type of shit that happens to other people. It's a little surreal, to be honest.

Writing this book has been a massive step in my healing process. Infertility is not something you get over, however. Like grief, it is a continual and ongoing process.

The lessons learned throughout my fertility journey have shaped my life, and who I am, in ways I can't even begin to describe.

Of course, there are things I wish I had done differently. Unfortunately, I can't go back in time and change things to make it easier for myself. However, I believe I was given this path to make it easier for those following in my footsteps.

So, I'm going to share all the things I learned along the way with you.

Let's start at the beginning of my journey. Approaching the expansion of your family in the same way you would undertake the development of a business plan is probably not the best strategy. Having a baby is not something that you can schedule in your planner. And while this attitude has served you well previously, it won't work here. Unfortunately having a baby does not work according to a schedule or timeline. Over planning when you're struggling to conceive will only lead to undue stress and disappointment. To survive, you must be willing to release the timeframe attached to WHEN this will happen. Smash the shit out of that biological clock that's ticking in your ear.

And while you're at it, remove the picture you have in your head of HOW things are supposed to turn out. Whether it's carrying a cup of sperm in your handbag or yelling at your husband that its GO time for sex, there will inevitably be times on this journey where you will shake your head and wonder where it all went so wrong. Make peace with your current path and accept that things may be a little different. Try to be flexible and pivot when you come across a roadblock instead of trying to run through it. The more you fight against it, the harder it will be. Detaching yourself from how and when it happens will ease the disappointment, and even out the ups and downs on this roller coaster.

Just because the road is rocky, doesn't mean you're not supposed to be a mum or that you'll be a terrible mum. We search high and low for a reason why this is happening to us. The truth is that there is no reason WHY. There is no reason why you're struggling to fall pregnant, yet Sally down the road is popping out kids like they're skittles. It isn't karma, you aren't being punished, and this is not your fault. I used to have the attitude that everything happens for a reason, so I lay awake at night, wondering why this was happening to us. What I do know is that we all have different paths, and searching high and low for a reason will sometimes guide you to the wrong conclusion. Too much bad shit happens in this world for there to be a reason for everything - but I do believe there is a lesson. Usually, you can't see it until after the storm is over, however.

Infertility is not something you can work at. I found that out the hard way. Hard work does not equal results. In fact, it can have the opposite effect. The harder you push, the more consumed you become, which increases your stress levels. And stress and infertility, as you know, do not mix.

I'm not saying sit on your ass and do nothing. There are things you can do to make sure you have the best chance of conceiving. But you should be doing all of those things anyway. Looking after your mind and body should be a priority regardless of whether you're trying to have a baby. Beyond that, you cannot control the outcome. And if you are a Type A personality like me who is used to getting what they want by working harder, this will hurt - a lot. You cannot control how many follicles are retrieved, you cannot control how many embryos are fertilised, and you sure as shit cannot control whether one or two lines appear on that stick. Take one day and one step at a time.

Let's talk about sex because that's what happens next. One of the biggest surprises on this journey was the impact it had on our sex life. I went into it thinking it would be fun to make a baby. But, when it became a source of failure, it took its toll on both my husband and I. The first thing you should know is that his resistance to sex and inability to perform is not about you. It isn't because he doesn't find you attractive or love you any less, it's because you're trying to schedule in something that should be spontaneous. When you march him into the bedroom demanding action, it not only sucks the romance and foreplay out of the situation, it puts additional pressure on him too. And just like stress affects your ability to conceive, it affects your partners' ability to perform.

Prioritise your mental and physical well-being NOW. Not when you get to the end. Now. How can you expect your body to make a baby, which requires a lot of energy when you're running on empty in every area of your life? I continually punished my body and pushed down my emotions because I just wanted to get to the end. I thought it would be over soon enough and that I could deal with the fallout later. I thought that all of the trauma would just fall away once I became a mum. But it doesn't, no matter how long you're on this roller coaster.

Because the truth is, when you get to the end, the grief doesn't magically disappear. And that's exactly what this is. We are grieving that picture we had in our head. We are grieving the loss of ourselves. We are grieving lost babies. The emotional scars don't go away until you face them. Don't push down your feelings and pretend to others and yourself that you're ok.

In order to heal, you must feel. And yes, that is so freaking difficult because the emotions and situations we're dealing with are so enormous that we can't even comprehend them most days. Because of that, your first reaction will be to bury your head in the sand and push the pain down inside you. You will focus on the next step, and the end goal to distract yourself from the devastation and anger you feel. Please don't do this. When you start burying the pain, you lose the ability to feel. And if you don't feel sadness, you won't experience joy. You will think more and feel less. That will form a bad habit that will spread into every corner of your life. If you don't feel, you won't endure as much pain; however, you will be numb. And being numb is no way to live. You didn't come this far only to live half a life. You deserve much more than that.

For seven years, I carried a lot of emotional baggage and undealt with emotions. It accumulated over time and was overwhelming and heavy. You need to lighten the load you're carrying. Being angry doesn't help - it's completely counter-productive. A lot of the time, we just look for the bandaid, or the quick fix, instead of focusing on the real problem - unpacking those emotions. Find something that will allow you to release the pain, negativity, frustration and doubts you've been holding onto. To let go of the stress and anxiety that's overwhelming you and take back control of your life. For some it is acupuncture, for some it's yoga, others it's running. This is one of the keys to being on this journey without it consuming you.

You don't have to prove to anyone or yourself that you are strong. Everyone knows it. Showing your emotions does not make you weak. I have always held the greatest admiration for those who aren't afraid of being vulnerable and showing their real feelings. I have learned that holding in your emotions is exhausting, and you can't be brave if you're tired. If you feel like crying.........cry. If you're angry....... yell. And you will be angry - a lot. You deserve to be mad because this does suck; just don't live there. Set yourself a time limit, throw yourself a pity party, then pick yourself up and move forward.

It is ok to take a break, to take a step back and regroup. I understand that you want to get off this roller coaster as soon as possible. Taking a pause doesn't mean that you're giving up, and it doesn't mean that you are weak. Reconnect with why you're doing this in the first place. Giving your mind and body a break may actually allow this to happen faster, and with less failed cycles. Because your body is always working for you. It knows what you need. And if you're physically and emotionally exhausted, it won't give you anything else to carry.

There aren't a finite number of babies to be allocated, and taking a month off doesn't mean that you'll miss out on your baby. It feels weird to write that, but our overthinking tells us that if we skip a cycle, this could be the one. We're scared that this may be the cycle our baby is coming, and because we didn't show up, our baby goes to someone else. It doesn't work that way.

Stop the comparison game. It's in our nature to compare our life with others. It's the reason why we are so triggered by seeing a pregnancy announcement or a pregnant woman in the street. We look at them and assume that because they have the one thing we crave; they must have a perfect life. Then we get angry because, well, why do they have it all? What looks like an easy life on the outside, however, may be opposite in reality. Accept that we all have different journeys and different forms of hard. This is your HARD.

And then the guilt starts. We feel guilty for feeling disappointed or jealous of others who have a more effortless path than us. We feel guilty for complaining when others have it worse than us. We feel guilty for wanting more.

The truth is, you do not need to feel guilty. Never minimise your feelings because things could always be worse. Yes, there are people out there who have it worse than you do, but there is no need to rank your emotions or feelings against others. Your feelings are entirely valid. Never feel guilty for wanting more. Sure, you should be grateful for what you have, but that doesn't mean you need to feel guilty because you want another baby, or because you wish it had happened a different way. And just because there are people who would love to be in your position, it doesn't mean we have to give up on our dreams. You are entitled to want more for your life. Don't let anyone tell you to settle. It is entirely possible to be grateful and want more at the same time.

There is a HUGE amount of literature and information out there. While it is good to be informed, overconsumption can drive you crazy. This process is overwhelming enough without you questioning every single decision you make. If it doesn't give you comfort or make you feel good, limit your intake.

There are so many statistics and averages thrown around on the internet, that it's hard not to get caught up in your odds. But understand that you are not a number, you are a person. Resist the temptation to put yourself in the average category. If I learned anything on this journey, it's that I am not average. And nor are you. And that's a good thing. It means that anything is possible. Getting consumed and scared by your chances is not serving you.

Just like me, you can be the exception to the rule. There are women all over the world who get pregnant naturally after 40. Who fall pregnant despite having endometriosis and polycystic ovarian syndrome. And most importantly, women who have unexplained infertility fall pregnant every single day. Don't let a doctor or a statistic tell you that this will not happen for you. Remove "this could never happen to me" from your vocabulary and go for it!

Your fertility specialist should be someone you trust. Don't be afraid to change if you don't feel heard or if you're not comfortable with them. You are in this together, working as a team. You need the right people in your corner. And you need people who believe in you.

And most importantly, trust your intuition. You know, that niggle in the pit of your stomach that pops up now and then? I know that it's tough to believe it when you're paralysed in fear of making the wrong decision - you just want your specialist to decide for you. Your doctors may be smart, but you know your body better than anyone else. Ask for the test, question the protocol, and don't be afraid to ask them to explain it to you over and over again. That's what you're paying them for.

Don't let anyone, including that voice in your head, tell you to give up on what you desire. If a baby is what you truly want, you can move mountains to get there. And when you don't think you can go any further, you can. When you believe there is no other way, there is. I never knew how strong or determined I was until infertility hit me.

I want to be clear, however, that NEVER GIVE UP is MY lesson. And it became a lesson for me because we ended our journey with two beautiful children. It may not be your lesson, however. I'm conscious of throwing out the advice of *"just don't give up"* because it gives the impression that walking away from your dream of having a baby is a sign of weakness. On the contrary, I believe it takes an incredible amount of strength to decide to choose YOU over expanding your family. My heart goes out to anyone who finds themselves at that fork in the road. Where they have to decide whether to keep pushing, despite it killing them from the inside out, or sacrifice their dream of becoming a mum to save themselves. It takes a level of bravery that I cannot even comprehend.

In my case, our approach of not giving up was the right one. I don't like to speculate on the scenario of when we would have walked away if things hadn't worked out how they did. We had spoken about what life would look like without children. But I am grateful that we didn't have to make that difficult decision.

Dealing with a miscarriage is a massive part of infertility. Most of us have had one, if not multiple. I find it heartbreaking that we usually minimise the loss. Whether we're being practical and saying that it wasn't a real baby anyway, or just not knowing how to deal with it, we usually push past it onto the next cycle. Firstly, it is ok to be devastated and feel empty. Take all the time you need to grieve. Secondly, and I cannot stress this enough; it is not your fault. There is very little that you can do yourself that will induce a miscarriage; however, we always search for what we did wrong and blame ourselves. And despite you feeling like you're the only one, you're not. You have nothing to feel embarrassed about, so talk to someone who has been through it too.

To hope or not to hope. This is something we all struggle with on this journey. Whenever we get our hopes up, and it doesn't happen, it bloody hurts. So, we associate the pain at the end, with the hope we feel at the beginning. And that causes us to go through every single cycle, thinking it isn't going to work, just to protect ourselves. Before each cycle ends, we think about the next one.

Hope is not the enemy. For me, hope is what got me through the darkest of hours. Hope is what will get you out of bed in the morning. Hope is what will push you forward time and time again. The disappointments will be just as painful, regardless of whether you hold hope or not. If you don't have hope, what is the point?

I believe that your mindset has an impact on the outcome too. What you focus on grows. So, if you approach life from a place of scarcity, lack and negativity, that is what you will manifest. Now before you jump to the conclusion that this is all your fault, take a pause here. This information is not to be used as a way to punish or blame yourself. But we do need to take responsibility for the part our thoughts, beliefs and mindset plays in any part of our life.

This doesn't mean going into every cycle faking hope and chanting affirmations that you don't believe. You'll just trigger your bullshit factor reflex and feel like a fraud. I'm talking about having faith and belief that this will all work out how it's supposed to in the end. Of course, it would be a lot easier knowing how your story ends while you're still in the journey, but that's not how life works. Approaching each cycle with faith and belief, as opposed to false hope, is a lot more digestible.

It's so easy to get caught up in our quest for a baby. Soon it becomes our only goal and sole focus. And the longer it takes, the more obsessed we get with it. We begin to confuse our failed attempts with who we are. And the more we intertwine our goal with our value, the more we sink into the self-limiting belief that we are not enough. That we need a baby to complete us.

Firstly, your value is not in your ability to have a child. You are enough right now. Your legacy begins and ends with you, not anyone else.

And secondly, you need to have something else to reach for aside from a baby. Your only goal cannot be to have a baby, because you're setting yourself up for failure. Distraction is essential for survival on this journey. Take up a new hobby, immerse yourself in a project that has nothing to do with cycles and hormones.

I know infertility seems like such a high mountain to climb. I know it feels like you've been trying to reach the top forever. And I know you can't see the summit through the clouds. But you won't feel like this forever. One day you will look back and be able to see that this is merely a chapter for you. This is not who you are, nor is this your whole story. There is so much more to your life than this small part.

Release your fears. Looking back on my journey, the number of fears I had was innumerable. But most of them were irrational and things I had made up in my head. I was giving them meaning and wasting my energy, giving them power when they didn't deserve any more than a shrug. I was scared of needles and overcame it. I was scared that all of our challenges meant I wouldn't be a good mum, and I am. I was afraid that this would all be for nothing, and it wasn't. I know you're scared. But at the end of the day, our fears are just thoughts. And because they are only thoughts, you get to choose them. Would you rather live in fear, or let them go and have faith?

Forgive people for not saying the right thing. I'm not saying that it's ok for them to ask you when you're going to have a baby, it's still an inappropriate question. But understand that they're not trying to make you feel bad on purpose. They don't know how painful it is to be asked that question, because they have not walked in your shoes. Their questions are based on their own experiences, and the truth is that they just don't know any better. I do believe we must educate and correct those people; however, because ignorance is no excuse for being insensitive. But do not hold onto the hate and resentment toward them - because hate is heavy, and you already have enough to carry.

You're in control of what you tell people. If you decide to tell them the truth about why you don't have children and it makes them feel uncomfortable, that's on them, not you. You are not responsible for other people's comfort.

Your family and friends are just trying to make you feel better by providing you with advice. And while it isn't helpful to hear about a friend of a friend who miraculously fell pregnant, or told to go on a holiday, they just want to take away your pain. And let's be honest, you have no idea how to make yourself feel better, nor do you have any idea what you need. So expecting others to say the right thing is setting them up for failure. Show them compassion and walk away.

Let go of what other people think. I was always so worried about people judging me for the lengths we went to for our babies. But at the end of the day, the only person that has to live with your decisions is you. This is your life. Unless they're in the trenches with you, other people don't get a say in your life. Other people's opinions of you are none of your business.

You are not alone. I know this journey can be lonely and isolating. It will seem like the whole world is against you, and you will want to scream at the injustice of it all. But I want you to know that you're not the only one that this is happening to. You don't have to travel this path in silence. Reach out to others who have been through the same thing and gain strength from their stories of survival, courage and success.

ACKNOWLEDGEMENTS

This book and our story would not be possible without the fantastic support and guidance of those closest to me.

First and foremost, thank you to Renee. How do you acknowledge someone who gave you a life? Without you, I would never have become a mother. You rode this roller coaster with us, never once complaining and getting back up after every knock-down. Thank you for teaching me that selfless angels are walking amongst us.

Of course, my husband, Craig. Thank you for walking through life with me, and being my partner in crime. For picking me up after every setback, sharing my anger and disappointment, and putting up with my erratic emotions and complete stubbornness. It hasn't always been easy, but I can't imagine travelling down this path with anyone else. Thank you for trusting me to follow my passion of helping others through infertility and allowing me to share our most intimate and darkest moments (including talking about your sperm and our sex life) in this book.

My two little miracles, Luca and Sophie. Thank you for choosing me to be your mummy. You were worth every tear, every penny, and every minute we had to wait.

To Nathan. This is an apology 10 years in the making. Thank you for the sacrifices you made so that we could have our family. I will be forever grateful.

My editor and good friend, Rebecca Patterson. Thank you for holding my hand as we walked through some of my darkest moments and for teaching me to acknowledge and identify the feelings I had pushed down for so long. For your gentle guidance, encouragement and generosity. You inspired so much healing, and I will treasure our deep (and somewhat tearful) conversations.

My friend and former life coach, Shannon Rose. Your belief in me planted a seed and set me on a path beyond my wildest dreams. I never knew true purpose, until you showed me yours. Thank you for asking the right questions.

To every single person who has been touched by infertility. I am in awe of your strength, bravery and determination. Thank you for inspiring me to show up every single day and continue to grow and heal so I can be the best damn coach and leader. I feel honoured to be a voice for those who aren't able to stand up for themselves, and raise awareness for an illness that is dripped in shame and miseducation.

ABOUT THE AUTHOR

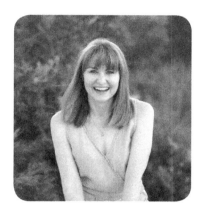 Jennifer Robertson is a fertility coach and has helped women all over the world to transform their mindset and take back control of their life in the midst of infertility.

Throughout her seven-year fertility journey, Jen discovered that her old ways of pushing and working hard weren't serving her. She is now using the lessons she learned along the way to develop programs and support those who are still struggling to conceive.

A former chief financial officer and your typical Type A, get shit done personality, Jen now lives by the beach with her husband and two beautiful children. She uses her experience and voice to raise awareness for a disease that affected her personally and continues to touch so many others around the world.

You can follow Jennifer on Instagram @msjenniferrobertson

Or contact her via her website – www.jenniferrobertson.co

Made in the USA
Las Vegas, NV
26 February 2023

68171014R00108